Well-Being: Expanding the Definition of Progress

THE ROBERT WOOD JOHNSON FOUNDATION CULTURE OF HEALTH SERIES

Series Editor, Alonzo L. Plough

Well-Being: Expanding the Definition of Progress

*Insights From Practitioners, Researchers, and
Innovators From Around the Globe*

EDITED BY ALONZO L. PLOUGH

OXFORD
UNIVERSITY PRESS

OXFORD
UNIVERSITY PRESS

Oxford University Press is a department of the University of Oxford. It furthers
the University's objective of excellence in research, scholarship, and education
by publishing worldwide. Oxford is a registered trade mark of Oxford University
Press in the UK and certain other countries.

Published in the United States of America by Oxford University Press
198 Madison Avenue, New York, NY 10016, United States of America.

Library of Congress Control Number: 2020935844

ISBN 978–0–19–008049–5

5 7 9 8 6 4

Printed by LSC Communications, United States of America

CONTENTS

SECTION VII   REFLECTIONS

FOREWORD

"What kind of ancestor do you want to be?"

What a profound question. I first heard it raised by Romlie Mokak, CEO of the Lowitja Institute, at a convening the Robert Wood Johnson Foundation (RWJF) hosted on well-being in Bellagio, Italy. Rom, a Djugun man and a member of the Yawuru people of Australia, explained that this inquiry serves as a guide when Indigenous communities consider important decisions.

It was an incredible way to begin our deliberation. I find that I am so often focused on the immediate outcome of our work that the idea of thinking about its impact across generations is at first disorienting, and then quite liberating. Asking this question introduces a different type of analysis, and a different meaning of "outcome."

At RWJF, we believe health means more than being free of disease. Since 1948, the World Health Organization has defined health as "a state of complete physical, mental, and social well-being and not merely the absence of disease or infirmity."[1] We support this definition, but we know it is not always the way health is defined in America.

We see exciting work happening around the globe. In many places, approaches to better health have moved beyond disease-specific measures, and the goal of societal well-being is being used to design innovative programs, to structure budgets, and to build community engagement. At RWJF, we have embraced a vision of working with others to build a national Culture of Health that advances overall well-being and equity. Our aim is to help ensure everyone has a fair and just opportunity to be as healthy as possible.

We know health is influenced by life experiences, social connections, and the current and historic barriers people may face—including racism, sexism, and other forms of discrimination. We know it is tied to where people live, learn, work, play, and pray. And one of the primary objectives of our work is to shift how people think about health.

Intrigued by what we might learn about health and well-being from around the globe, RWJF brought together 32 thought leaders representing 19 countries and a range of disciplines for a gathering in September 2018 at the Rockefeller Foundation Bellagio Conference Center in Italy. The group included researchers and academics; policymakers; leaders from civic, grassroots, and private-sector organizations; and other leaders with diverse and complementary perspectives. (Please see the full list of participants at the back of the book.) Most had not met each other before, and many remarked on how refreshing it was to attend a meeting with a new group and different perspectives. The one thing everyone had in common was an eagerness to advance well-being and embed it into the social, economic, and cultural fabrics of their nations and communities.

Rom's question deeply resonated with the meeting participants, and it set the stage for open and productive discussions: How might a focus on future generations steer conversations about equity, justice, resilience, and sustainability? How does it affect the way we think about health today as well as tomorrow?

This book provides ideas and guidance on advancing well-being locally, nationally, and internationally. And it illuminates how diverse communities and cultures can work together to strengthen these efforts.

It's my hope that these insights will help us all continue to ask—and answer—the question, "What kind of ancestors do we want to be?"

—Richard E. Besser, MD
President and Chief Executive Officer
Robert Wood Johnson Foundation
United States

Introduction

The Imperative for Well-Being in an Inequitable World

KARABI ACHARYA, SCD, MHS
Director, Global Ideas for U.S. Solutions,
Robert Wood Johnson Foundation, United States

ALONZO L. PLOUGH, PHD, MPH, MA
Chief Science Officer and Vice President, Research-Evaluation-Learning,
Robert Wood Johnson Foundation, United States

How would the world change if we made policy, resource, and other decisions not based solely on short-term targets, like growing the economy or preventing specific diseases, but to achieve long-term well-being for all people, communities, and the environment?

Certainly, this includes vast improvements in physical health, economic stability, and basic needs. But it also includes improved social connections and a sense of belonging and purpose. It includes more moments of joy and happiness, as well as a deeper sense of satisfaction with life. It emphasizes equity and human rights, and the interconnection among people and between people and planet. The question for this book is how are people, communities, and countries around the world pursuing these goals? What are the policies and programs that they have put into place? How do they talk about what really matters? How do they know if they're on the path toward well-being?

The answers to these questions signal a potential shift in how we understand the human condition, how we define progress locally and globally, and how we ensure opportunities for people to thrive in every aspect of life and to create meaningful futures.

This is the idea behind using a well-being framework to define, pursue, and measure progress, an approach that is gaining currency around the world. (See

Figure on page xiv for an overview of the components of a well-being framework.) It offers:

- *Equity focus:* At its core, increasing well-being requires changing power dynamics, including a far more diverse set of voices and communities in decision-making, and advancing more equitable opportunities and outcomes. One of the fundamental benefits of using well-being as a definition of progress is that it builds in increasing equity (ensuring that everyone has what they need) and addressing inequities (unfair, avoidable differences in opportunity) as a core goal and driver for policy and practice choices. And the process of applying a well-being approach brings transparency to the indicators that are measured and outcomes that are tracked.
- *A more human-centered view of how things are going:* A well-being lens—drawing on both objective data and subjective, or self-reported, measures—illuminates the people behind the numbers and reveals clues that are not apparent in disease data or economic indicators alone. Deaths from opioid addiction might be predicted by population-level data on isolation, worry, and despair. Climate change is not just about disagreement on quantitative predictions of temperature rise, but also the current inequitable impact of extreme weather on the health of marginalized communities.
- *Holistic approaches:* By illuminating interconnected physical, psychological, social, cultural, political, economic, and ecological factors, a well-being framework surfaces needs that cannot be addressed by single sectors or academic fields. Addressing equity and improving well-being become fundamental parts of every decision, not relegated to the equity team or the human rights commission. As opposed to separating issues into housing or health care or other needs, a well-being approach looks at interconnections and outcomes.
- *Interconnectedness:* A well-being approach brings to the forefront the mutuality and interdependence of our lives and societies, illuminating how the well-being of any one of us is linked with the well-being of others, the community's well-being overall, and the well-being of the natural world. It recognizes the need to move away from the notion of purely individual "success"—which is so ingrained in U.S. culture as to be almost reflexive—and embrace the value of relational well-being.

Our world is in the midst of unprecedented challenges—from the impacts of climate change and the humanitarian crisis of forced migration, to the rise of nationalism and epidemic growth of deaths of despair; the COVID-19 pandemic and global demands for anti-racism are deeply intertwined with all of these issues. These challenges require new approaches catalyzing communities, cities, and countries around the globe to embrace a well-being framework to assess progress and guide solutions.

"As we reflect on the past decade of political and economic upheaval," said Nicola Sturgeon, first minister of Scotland, "of growing inequalities, and when we look ahead to the challenges of the climate emergency, increasing automation, an aging population, then I think the argument for the case for a much broader definition of what it means to be successful as a country, as a society, is compelling, and increasingly so."[1]

The shift Sturgeon is describing is reshaping Scotland's government. Similar shifts are afoot from New Zealand to Santa Monica, Calif.; from Nova Scotia to Singapore. It's an idea born in Bhutan in the 1970s of Buddhist principles and a commitment to human flourishing and prosperity. It's been molded over time, drawing on psychology, anthropology, neuroscience, sociology, public health, and many other disciplines, and honed by economists, policymakers, and innovative practitioners on the ground. It's reflected in broad, goal-setting progress measures, such as the Sustainable Development Goals (SDGs) and Environmental, Social, and Governance criteria (ESGs), proof that the old ways of thinking are no longer sufficient.

Despite this momentum, many governments, international bodies, and the dominant narratives that inform how people view the world continue to define progress by largely economic measures. Not surprisingly, this leads to policies and practices focused disproportionately on consumption. This continued dominance of economic-based decisions has failed to help us understand or make progress on increases in inequity, erosion of social capital, and unfair opportunities for intergenerational prosperity.

To be certain, this is not merely about one set of measures or another. Much of the global conversation about well-being frameworks and approaches to date has focused on the false dichotomy of moving "beyond GDP." This book invites a much more nuanced conversation about defining, pursuing, and measuring progress based on a significantly broader set of indicators. Well-being indicators, inclusive of and in concert with economic indicators, have the potential to be this new compass.

As Richard Besser notes in his foreword, a well-being approach also has the potential to expand the conception of health, moving far beyond tracking diseases, identifying causes, and developing treatments, vaccines, and prevention strategies. As a foundation committed to a national agenda to build a Culture of Health* in America, we are focused on the social determinants of health—those

---

* The Foundation is dedicated to building a Culture of Health that provides everyone in America a fair and just opportunity for health and well-being. This requires removing obstacles to health such as poverty, discrimination, and their consequences, including powerlessness and lack of access to good jobs with fair pay, quality education and housing, safe environments, and health care.

A Framework for Understanding Human Well-Being

Objective Well-Being

Measures of objective well-being often use administrative and survey-based data to quantify and describe assets and occurrences at each level. These are:

- Based on predetermined criteria and often performed by external observation.
- Used to document phenomena that exist independent of subjective awareness, though not divorced from subjective value judgment.

Examples include:*

- Evidence of inclusion or participatory democracy
- Historical context (e.g., institutional inequity)
- GDP

- Number, quality, density, and use of built features, like parks or roads
- Crime rates
- Cultural norms and narratives

- Household income
- Incidence of clinical outcomes or care utilization rates
- Social connections

*Indicators listed within each realm are examples of the types of data that may help define well-being; they are not exhaustive.

Civic Well-Being
Governance and Policies

Community Well-Being
Status, Amenities, Culture

Individual Well-Being

Developed by Trené Hawkins, RWJF, with collaboration and input from Anita Chandra, RAND Corporation, and Carol Graham, the Brookings Institution.

Subjective Well-Being

Measures of subjective well-being are usually collected at the individual level and generally describe satisfaction with or perception of features, behaviors, and events at the civic, community, and individual levels. This includes direct assessment (e.g., survey) or more passive monitoring (e.g., social media).

- **Evaluative** measures reflect an assessment of an individual's life as a whole and their satisfaction with it.
- **Eudaimonic** metrics express individual perceptions of meaning and purpose in their lives.
- **Hedonic** metrics are binary and measure individual emotional or affective states, such as feelings of pleasure or pain.
- **Flourishing** is often used to describe the ultimate outcome of subjective well-being.

Examples include:*

- Trust in government or perceived corruption

Civic Well-Being
Governance and Policies

- Satisfaction with quality or aesthetic of community features or impact on participation in desired activities
- Perceived safety

Community Well-Being
Status, Amenities, Culture

- Ability to make choices about the direction of one's life course
- Access to health care and education
- Social connections/friendships

Individual Well-Being

Often represent the state of the larger ecosystem (including natural systems) and its impact on well-being; can include measures of sustainability but also measures of environmental health and quality independent of potential to serve human needs.

Well-Being of Environment and Planet

social, economic, and environmental conditions that influence individual and group health status. A well-being framework considers all of this, and then poses even higher-order questions about the aspiration and goals of human society. Again, we're not looking to replace one idea with another. Rather, we're eager to learn what's happening in places where there is an intentional effort to advance well-being constructs and to define progress more broadly.

This sense of inquiry, curiosity, and the great potential to adopt promising practices from around the world inspired us to convene the group at Bellagio. Our goal: to advance global dialogue and action on the well-being construct, and to inform RWJF's work with others to create a Culture of Health in the United States. We were particularly interested in learning how to apply a well-being approach to advance health equity in radically different settings, looking for clues about potential practices to use in a country like ours with very diverse populations and contexts.

The conversation at Bellagio—and in this book—focuses on moving beyond how to define and measure well-being, a topic that receives significant global attention. It explores how cities and countries are applying well-being data and concepts as a driver for action; informing practice shifts, policy and systemic change, and resource allocation; and ultimately creating a new definition of what matters. It's recognition that a well-being approach is more than a measurement of human conditions; it is a way of thinking, understanding, and taking action. As Jacinda Ardern, prime minister of New Zealand and champion for her country's well-being budget, put it: "We're fundamentally changing the way we do policymaking to make sure that we deliver on well-being, not just economic success."[2]

Overview of the Book

This book, the fourth in RWJF's Culture of Health series, uses a call-and-response format in each section to mirror the conversations at Bellagio. Each section begins with a paper prepared by participants before the conference, followed by a chapter with insights that emerged during discussion of those papers and many other topics. The chapters draw heavily on case studies presented by five of the practitioners at Bellagio to share their on-the-ground learnings. Full write-ups of the cases appear in Section VI to illustrate the dynamics, nuances, and complexity of how a well-being approach plays out in a range of very different contexts. The resulting volume, then, is a collection of distinct voices and ideas, at times academic and at times ruggedly practical, encompassing both stand-alone sections and themes that weave throughout every chapter.

Among those recurring themes are both alignment and corroboration of ideas, as well as some contradiction or discrepancy. This is not surprising since we quite intentionally brought different voices and perspectives to the conversation, and it underscores both the emergent nature of this field as well as the variety of well-being approaches shaped by cultural context and reality. We hope this range of opinions will spark your own thinking and invite you to see the many angles and possibilities of this work.

The participants made it clear that there is no *single* way to advance well-being; there is no *one* well-being framework, approach, or construct. Our gathering did not aim to reach consensus or create a directive, so this book is neither a recipe nor a prescription. We are not here to assess or label which efforts are "full well-being" and which reflect individual elements of a well-being approach. Rather, the hope is that sharing this thinking will help others craft solutions that are relevant in their communities and that spark transformative action.

The sections include:

- **Section I, "Why Well-Being,"** makes the case for centering decision-making, resource allocation, and cultural expectations on well-being. It considers whether a well-being frame can advance our equity strategies more rapidly.
- **Section II, "Defining Well-Being and Indicators of Progress,"** looks at the role of measurement in advancing well-being approaches and improving individual and collective well-being, and why the "dials on the dashboard" matter. It then explores the power that measures have to create shifts in narrative, practice, and policy.
- **Section III, "Narratives and Culture,"** explores the need for a new narrative, the collection of stories that help people make sense of the world and form ideas of "how things are." Shifting the narrative from predominantly "wealth and economic growth matter most" to recognizing that "well-being is our end goal" creates the opportunity to fundamentally change expectations, decisions, and equitable outcomes. This section also delves into the role of cultural context in defining and advancing well-being.
- **Section IV, "Learning From Other Movements and the Need to Shift Power,"** explores how well-being approaches must be designed by the community and engage and build power—not merely representation—among people who are often excluded from decision-making, including Indigenous peoples, youth, people living with lower incomes, and women.
- **Section V, "Breaking Down Silos and Encouraging Innovation,"** begins in the public sector, examining how the more comprehensive framework of well-being can motivate cross-sector approaches and cross-cutting solutions. It then explores roles for different sectors and opportunities to align with other movements.
- **Section VI, "Case Studies,"** provides detailed reports of approaches, results, and lessons from five diverse contexts.
- **Section VII, "Reflections,"** includes the perspectives of two U.S. thought leaders—one a practitioner, the other an academic—on the promise of

well-being approaches and the opportunity for ongoing learning and evolution. We also share insights about what this has sparked in our thinking, and outline some of RWJF's own efforts and plans ahead.

A Time for Inquiry, Reflection, and Action

Above all, this book invites you into the rich dialogue and spirit of inquiry at Bellagio. It brings you into the questions that started this journey: What would our communities be like if every decision was made to improve well-being for all? What would have to shift first? As we continue to explore efforts from South Africa to Canada to Paraguay, how do we apply what we learn to build well-being in East Baltimore, in West Texas, in Southeast Alaska, and everywhere in between? It invites you to ask: How can these insights inform and inspire the regions and sectors where I work and the decisions I influence?

We live in a time where significant, interconnected challenges require that we shift our definitions and pursuit of progress to go much further upstream and to make fundamental changes. The global work of advancing well-being offers potential to make significant impact. We hope you will read this book, find ideas and approaches that resonate and can advance your own work, and are inspired to advance well-being in an inequitable world.

WHY WELL-BEING

As highlighted in the introduction and detailed throughout this book, a global discussion is taking place about the potential to broaden the definition of progress to encompass well-being. Two fundamental ideas that permeated the discourse at Bellagio were the fact that shifting to a well-being approach will both require and result in a real focus on increasing equity; and that there are incredible potential benefits to people, communities, and the planet when decisions are made with the goal of advancing well-being.

Chapter 1, *Well-Being as a Pathway to Equity,* dives headlong into the first idea, weaving together three papers prepared by Bellagio participants to set the stage for the meeting. It explores three inequities that matter the most in terms of impact on well-being—income inequality, threats to human rights, and gaps in social cohesion—and how a well-being framework offers new potential to understand and address those and other inequities. It also discusses whether a well-being frame can create a broad opportunity to engage policymakers and stakeholders across a diverse political spectrum in discussions of equity.

Chapter 2, *The Rationale for a Well-Being Approach: Discussion and Case Studies From Bellagio,* touches on both the frank discussion of the challenges of a well-being approach, and the incredible excitement and optimism about its potential. At scale, this work has the potential to significantly transform systems, structures, and cultural expectations, and to deliver tangible benefits to people, communities, the environment, and future generations. Some benefits that resonated across the group—spanning boundaries of fields, cultural contexts, and worldviews—included fostering collaboration and holistic action, taking an intergenerational approach, linking people and planet, and helping to change public narratives and expectations about what people value in their societies.

Well-Being as a Pathway to Equity

Based on papers prepared for the Bellagio gathering by:

WALTER FLORES, PHD
*Executive Director, Center for the Study of Equity and
Governance in Health Systems, Guatemala*

ÉLOI LAURENT, PHD
*Senior Economist, Sciences Po Centre for Economic Research,
France; and Visiting Professor, Stanford University, United States*

JENNIFER PRAH RUGER, PHD, MSC, MSL, MA
*Amartya Sen Professor of Health Equity, Economics and Policy,
School of Social Policy and Practice and Perelman School of
Medicine, University of Pennsylvania, United States*

In a world without equity, well-being is impossible. Inequities in income, health, education, environmental conditions, access to opportunity, and other factors hinder individual, community, and civic well-being. Pursuing a well-being approach centered on equity—from what gets measured and how, to the way stories are told and the voices that tell them, to what gets prioritized and acted upon and by whom—can reduce these inequities. And in the symbiotic relationship between well-being and equity, as well-being improves, so does equity; likewise, as equity improves so does well-being.

This chapter explores the link between well-being and equity, and makes the case for well-being approaches as a powerful pathway to advance equity. It is based on briefing papers by the authors listed above, who are researchers exploring indicators, conditions, and approaches to well-being from different perspectives. In their writing, these authors addressed three intersecting components of well-being and equity: economic equity, human rights, and social cohesion. Through these lenses, they explore implications and opportunities for social and policy change, suggest ways that it is possible to advance equity using a well-being approach, and illuminate work that remains to be done.

Please note that throughout this paper, and the book, we are using RWJF's definition of health equity: *Health equity means that everyone has a fair and just opportunity to live a healthier life no matter who they are, where they live, or how much money they make.* Equity is about access or opportunity, as opposed to equality, which is about outcomes and often means that everyone gets the same thing. In some cases, writers used the term equality in a way that mirrors the Foundation's definition of equity; we have maintained their language in direct quotes but changed to equity as relevant in all other uses.

Inequality Economics Make the Case for a Well-Being Approach

In the United States and comparable countries, income inequality leads to health problems, including higher rates of obesity, drug abuse, and mental illness. It can hinder economic dynamism and development, and is detrimental to resilience and long-term well-being. Without equity, it is more difficult for communities to deal with disasters such as hurricanes and terrorist attacks, ongoing stress and trauma, and ecological shocks, such as climate change.

> *Inequality leads to lower health outcomes in many ways.*
>
> —*Éloi Laurent*
> *Senior Economist*
> *Sciences Po Centre for Economic Research*
> *France*

"The lens of income inequality is the most successful strategy in shifting the debate from growth and GDP to well-being," says Éloi Laurent, senior economist at the Sciences Po Centre for Economic Research in France. Focusing on well-being illuminates inequities that can be masked in economic averages and indicators.

Over the last 30 years, income inequality *within* countries has grown, says Laurent. While income inequality *between* countries recently decreased, when combined with within-country inequality, overall income inequality has increased. The top 1 percent has gotten richer while the income of the bottom 50 percent has stalled. However, this growing gap in income inequality has been overlooked because of improvements in average well-being in areas such as health and education, and a persistent focus on economic growth and efficiency.

Along with the increase in income inequality, public understanding of income inequality has grown and interest in inequity economics has been renewed. Thomas Piketty put well-being at the center of public debate by shifting from the complicated Gini index (a summary measure of income inequality) to something people can easily understand: the share of the national income in the U.S. owned by the top 10 percent. Piketty's work, including his bestseller, *Capital in the Twenty-First Century* (2014), is the most visible sign of renewed interest in inequality economics.[1]

> *Health is a much more powerful metric of well-being than income inequality.*
> —*Éloi Laurent*
> *Senior Economist*
> *Sciences Po Centre for Economic Research*
> *France*

But income inequality, cautions Laurent, is economics in disguise. "It's economics criticizing economics, and it's only one aspect of human well-being." Laurent (and all other Bellagio participants) repeatedly underscored that the focus on economic metrics and economic growth as the sole path to success for all people masks other critical inequities. Further, economic metrics such as GDP, household income, and the Gini index are designed from the Western economic and social perspective. Developed using a top-down approach, without involving communities and individuals, they ignore indicators valued by Indigenous people and other communities, as well as the impact of historic and structural exclusion, racism, oppression, and marginalization.

For Indigenous people in Australia, Latin America, New Zealand, and North America, for example, the well-being of the natural environment is a key part of individual and community "wealth" and well-being, says Walter Flores, executive director of the Center for the Study of Equity and Governance in Health Systems, based in Guatemala and working globally.

Environmental Inequity and Well-Being

This link between human and planetary well-being raises another critical component of equity: environmental inequity. "Environmental conditions are not evenly distributed, and the notion of environmental inequality is crucial in understanding the impact of air pollution or climate change on human health," Laurent said. Equity influences communities' ability to organize efficiently, both to sustainably use natural resources and to resist ecological shocks, such as climate change.[2] This underscores the importance of environmental conditions for well-being and what Laurent describes as the "justice-sustainability nexus linking equality, well-being, and sustainability."

Some people are exposed to more pollution and environmental risks while others have more access to natural resources (water, clean air, and food) and amenities. Environmental justice aims to create equity by identifying, measuring, and correcting these environmental inequalities. Further, many scholars argue that societies will be more just if they are more sustainable and more sustainable if they are more just.[3-5] For example, consider two recent texts grounded in native culture and religious ethics:

- The 2010 Cochabamba Declaration from the World People's Conference on Climate Change states: "It is imperative that we forge a new system that restores harmony with nature and among human beings."[6]
- In 2015, Pope Francis wrote in *Laudato Si*': "We are faced not with two separate crises, one environmental and the other social, but rather with one complex crisis that is both social and environmental."[7]

> *It makes environmental sense to mitigate our social crisis and social sense to mitigate our environmental crises.*
>
> —*Éloi Laurent*
> *Senior Economist*
> *Sciences Po Centre for Economic Research*
> *France*

A well-being approach makes the inequities of environmental justice more visible while removing the false dichotomy and separation of human needs and environmental needs by incorporating ecosystem health and sustainability with human flourishing.

Establishing Well-Being as a Human Right

> *Human flourishing involves individuals being able to be and do what they want to be and do, reaching their full potential.*
>
> —*Jennifer Prah Ruger*
> *Amartya Sen Professor of Health Equity, Economics and Policy*
> *University of Pennsylvania*
> *United States*

Turning to another aspect of equity, human rights, Jennifer Prah Ruger, Bellagio participant and Amartya Sen professor of health equity, economics and policy at the University of Pennsylvania, makes the case that having enough to flourish, or achieving sufficiency, is a key expectation of both well-being and human rights. "Human flourishing and capabilities form a basis for a definition of well-being," she says. Well-being metrics help illuminate the differences between actual and potential functioning—and in so doing, spotlight injustices and opportunities to address them in the context of societal progress. With human flourishing and capabilities serving as a foundation for human rights, well-being can be framed as a human right. Thus, governments can be held accountable for ensuring well-being along with the more well-known human rights of health and standards of living.

The World Health Organization defines health inequities as "systematic differences in the health status of different population groups" that "have significant social and economic costs both to individuals and societies."[8] A focus on well-being and related policy actions can prevent avoidable health inequities. Well-being, says Laurent, "stems from an eternal and universal human question: What are the real drivers of human development and flourishing besides material conditions? What is a good life?"

Human rights are a policy lever for advancing well-being.
—*Jennifer Prah Ruger*
Amartya Sen Professor of Health Equity, Economics and Policy
University of Pennsylvania
United States

Identifying and then assessing a sufficiency threshold for well-being—everyone has enough—in a country will demonstrate inequities in well-being and other human rights. This, in turn, will enable development of policies to create conditions that allow all individuals to achieve sufficiency. Bhutan, which introduced the concept of Gross National Happiness (GNH) in the 1970s, is already focusing on sufficiency. The country's National GNH Survey assesses how many people reach a sufficiency threshold across different indicators of well-being. The Centre for Bhutan Studies and GNH Research and the GNH Commission analyze survey data across subgroups such as gender and rural/ urban areas. Policy and actions then focus on improving well-being for people who are falling below the sufficiency threshold.

Defining Human Rights in a Well-Being Context

Just as well-being indicators illuminate the stories behind economic data, health statistics, and other measures, they can also clarify the nature and scope of human rights beyond merely legal and institutional arrangements. "Well-being can be helpful in addressing ethical and practical debates in human rights," Prah Ruger says. "It can be an ethical and moral grounding of human rights. The system of rights is one variable that impacts well-being."

Well-being provides an analytical framework for understanding and evaluating human rights. An example of this framework shared in the discussion at Bellagio was that in Palestine, most people have spent their lives in warlike conditions. The trauma they experience includes shootings, tear gas, sound bombs, body and house searches, humiliation, insecurity, distress, uncertainty, verbal abuse, racism, and violation of basic rights, such as the right of movement of people and goods. New indicators related to suffering and human rights abuses, such as humiliation, human insecurity, and deprivation, have a demonstrated association with well-being.

More specifically, legally-binding international documents (e.g., the International Convention on the Elimination of Discrimination Against Women, the United Nations Convention on the Rights of the Child, the United Nations Convention Against Torture, and the International Convention on the Elimination of All Forms of Racial Discrimination) have codified basic ideas of equity, liberty, and dignity, as well as specific human rights, including:

- individual rights, such as the right to life
- prohibition of slavery
- freedom of thought, opinion, religion, conscience, association, and movement
- social, economic, and cultural rights
- rights to standards of living (food, clothing, housing, and social services) and health

Some of these rights are used as metrics to assess equity and well-being, such as adequate education. Governments are duty-bound to uphold human rights, *including well-being if it is framed as a human right.* Holding governments accountable for well-being as a human right is an approach to address inequities—so long as accountability extends to all populations.

In New Zealand, the Living Standards Framework helps government agencies consider a range of well-being dimensions that impact on human rights and freedom when planning and taking action. The Treasury plans to use quantitative data from well-being measures to shine light on the distribution of capital and resources across population groups. Data will be used to stimulate public discussion of which elements of well-being are most important to the people of New Zealand.

Inclusion, Social Cohesion, and Well-Being

Inclusion—taking part in society and having access to institutions and resources, including health and education—plays a vital role in equity, social justice, and power relations, creating space and shifting influence to different leaders, cultures, and views. Social cohesion is especially important. According to the Organisation for Economic Co-operation and Development,[9] "A cohesive society works toward the well-being of all of its members, minimizing disparities and avoiding marginalization." Cohesive societies can work to advance social justice and to shift power relations as they are more likely to:

- support relationship networks, trust, and identity among groups
- fight discrimination, exclusion, and excessive inequities
- enable upward social mobility

> *Inclusion and social cohesion are related under the umbrella of thriving for a better life for the individual, the family, the communities, and the society.*
> —*Walter Flores*
> *Executive Director*
> *Center for the Study of Equity and Governance in Health Systems*
> *Guatemala*

Benefits of social cohesion encompass many accepted indicators of well-being, including:

- more stable democracies and more civic participation
- more productivity, growth, and resilience in the face of economic problems
- better quality of life
- more inclusivity and tolerance of diversity and multiculturalism
- stronger conflict management and resolution
- better health outcomes, especially outcomes related to the links between health and income inequality, employment, and social support

"Well-being and social cohesion are interrelated," says Flores. An assessment of 27 European Union countries showed that people in more cohesive societies are happier and psychologically healthier. The Council of Europe identified providing access to employment, housing, social protection, health, and education as policy areas to improve inclusion and social cohesion.

Despite the benefits of inclusion and social cohesion for well-being, Flores offers several cautions. First, social cohesion can be exclusionary or can ignore diverse cultural values if it is focused on advancing dominant culture social norms. Highly cohesive societies may be closed off to minority groups and migrants, and may not value and respect their cultural assets.

A serious global discourse on social cohesion and well-being must address the risks of well-being becoming a Western agenda that ignores the historic and structural determinants of exclusion, oppression, and marginalization of some population groups.

—*Walter Flores*
Executive Director
Center for the Study of Equity and Governance in Health Systems
Guatemala

In Australia, for example, self-determination is central to well-being for the Indigenous people. The United Nations' Declaration on the Rights of Indigenous Peoples (2007) affirmed this as a key right. Despite this, government policies continuously ignore it and instead place an emphasis on social services, security, and other indicators—policies that appear to gently steer Indigenous Australians to adopt a Western style of life rather than providing them with opportunities to live lives of personal meaning and value as Indigenous peoples.[10]

"Social cohesion and well-being appear as top-down approaches," says Flores. "This seems to be at odds with the central goal of well-being, which includes participation in society, access to institutions and decisions over one's plan for life."

Additionally, cohesion within specific population groups or geographical areas may contradict values, norms, and laws set at the national level. For instance, a traditional community may be highly cohesive based on beliefs and practices that assign a lesser social role to members of the community (i.e., women or elderly).[11] This challenge is particularly important for countries with diverse ethnicity, says Flores.

It is also imperative to consider social justice and power relations as part of inclusion, social cohesion, and well-being, says Flores, but these concepts are too often left out of the well-being literature. "This is a major gap," he says, "especially when considering well-being for multi-ethnic societies, societies with Indigenous populations and a history of colonialism and social marginalization."

Ensuring That Well-Being Indicators Support Increased Equity

Designed with a clear commitment to illuminating and addressing inequities and advancing human rights, a well-being approach can be a powerful pathway to increasing equity. It has the potential to make addressing inequity visible—and accountable—in the policymaking process and provide data that can be used in determining priorities and making decisions about policies and budgets.

> *Indicators must not only change the way we see the world, but also help us change the way we conduct policy.*
>
> —*Éloi Laurent*
> *Senior Economist*
> *Sciences Po Centre for Economic Research*
> *France*

The ultimate goal is to enable conditions in which all people have a fair chance to flourish and reach their full potential. "The basic course of action is to make visible what matters for humans and then make it count," says Laurent. Individuals and communities must be engaged in defining indicators. Key players in developing and implementing the well-being approach must deeply listen to communities.

As is discussed throughout this book, well-being indicators are most powerful when they are applied to influence policy and action. A key example that Laurent calls out is integrating well-being and inequity indicators in budget procedures to reform policy. Currently, he says, politicians make budget decisions based on very little knowledge of the state of countries apart from aggregate macroeconomic indicators (such as GDP). The United Nations Sustainable Development Goals (SDGs) provide an example of integrating well-being and inequity indicators into the budget process: About 23 countries are integrating or have integrated the SDGs into their budget process, making addressing inequity a core part of their approach.

Well-Being and Equity: The Path Ahead

A well-being approach provides a new framework to address inequities in income, health, education, and environmental conditions, and for redefining—in an inclusive way—what matters most to individuals and communities. Widespread acceptance of well-being as a way to measure and pursue progress creates an opportunity to engage all stakeholders and decision-makers, especially those who might not come to the table for an equity-focused discourse.

> *What we're really after is the common good and the sense of connectedness that we all have with each other and with nature.*
>
> —*Jennifer Prah Ruger*
> *Amartya Sen Professor of Health Equity, Economics and Policy*
> *University of Pennsylvania*
> *United States*

Laurent, Prah Ruger, and Flores suggest some key considerations for the work ahead, including:

- Identifying leading, easy-to-understand indicators of well-being that make inequity visible, are the most understandable and impactful in the public debate, are integrated in an efficient narrative, and can be translated into policy change.
- Shifting from economic-only narratives of progress to narratives informed by well-being values and outcomes—which may expand opportunity for discourse about equity issues with those for whom inequity frames are triggers for "redistribution" or "taking."
- Clarifying which dimensions of well-being should be viewed as human rights.
- Further exploring the role of well-being in linking health and sustainability: Does it make environmental sense to mitigate the inequity crisis and ethical sense to mitigate environmental crises?
- Integrating equity indicators in policy and budgeting.
- Developing effective policies and programs to promote social inclusion, especially for marginalized populations, as a core element of well-being.
- Truth-telling, recognition, discussion, and actions to address historic practices, the racism of today, and the trauma experienced due to systematized oppression.

Well-being can be a powerful pathway to advance equity, so that all people everywhere have the opportunity and skills to lead meaningful lives. Applying well-being data and concepts can drive action, and inform policy change, system change, and resource allocation to focus on what matters most.

The Rationale for a Well-Being Approach

Discussion and Case Studies From Bellagio

A well-being approach—that is, establishing well-being as the goal and measure of what matters in order to create a future in which people, communities, and the planet can all thrive—provides a new compass for decision-making, resource allocation, social narrative, and even consciousness. The arrow points to a more comprehensive notion of health, one that focuses not only on disease prevention, but on creating the best opportunity to thrive in all aspects of life. It points away from the idea that money and consumption are the only pathways to progress, and toward a more holistic view of what matters. It shows how policies and actions affect people and communities differently, illuminating unique needs and gaps instead of being satisfied with aggregate numbers. "The focus on inequity [in well-being] is important because that brings in assessment, evaluation, and notions of justice, which is, there's something wrong with this picture," says Bellagio participant Jennifer Prah Ruger, Amartya Sen professor of health equity, economics and policy at the University of Pennsylvania.

By defining progress differently—designing new measures of what matters informed by people across the community and building aligned practices, policies, and actions—cities, nations, and society at large can radically expand the definition and pursuit of progress and create more equitable and environmentally-sound conditions.

We all share the feeling that being human, enjoying a good life, and enjoying good health is more than just money and more than just disease. So let's work together.

—Carrie Exton
Head of Section for Monitoring Well-Being and Progress
Organisation for Economic Co-operation and Development
France

The conversations at Bellagio, informed by diverse perspectives spanning geography, perspective, and sector, illustrated the potential for ideas, actions, policies, and authentic engagement of diverse stakeholders that, when combined, can create a powerful pathway to advance well-being and equity. "We're all critical and we're all calling for change," says Bellagio participant Rita Giacaman, professor at Birzeit University's Institute of Community and Public Health in Palestine. "And that's very good. But what I think is also important is the realization that we are not alone."

> *I look around and I see so many similarities—not only from southern countries but others as well. But to create change, what we need to do is get together and organize. And this is the first step in doing that. We give power to each other.*
> —Rita Giacaman
> *Professor, Institute of Community and Public Health*
> *Birzeit University*
> *Palestine*

Well-Being Benefits and Outcomes

Across the conversations at Bellagio, participants repeatedly highlighted the benefits, positive outcomes, and potential for transformation via a well-being approach. Some of the key points, further explored in this chapter and throughout the book, include the ability of a well-being approach to:

- **Shift the focus to things that matter most to people and communities**, deeply informed by grassroots engagement.
- **Create more urgency to address inequities and shift power** by illuminating conditions often masked by other measures and aggregate data.
- **Break down structural barriers and "silos" to encourage cross-sector collaboration.**
- **Link human well-being and environmental sustainability.**
- **Create a new expectation, demand, and accountability for a well-being approach** and a more equitable concept of progress.
- **Focus on the future** through long-term agendas and intergenerational leadership.

Focusing on what matters most

Well-being measures and practices have a unique ability to focus on and quantify essential elements of life that are left out of purely economic frameworks and other models. For example, Bellagio participants discussed the importance of human potential, cultural pride, and sense of purpose as crucial indicators of and goals for progress. These elements are front and center in Nova Scotia, where efforts are underway to replace the deficit-based story of sluggish economic and demographic growth with a mindset of abundance, based on the province's natural beauty, strong sense of community, high levels of education, and satisfaction with life. This asset-based definition of progress and community identity has the potential to buoy a new sense of collective optimism and inform programs and policies that build on Nova Scotia's positive attributes.

> *We lack clarity and confidence about our place in the world, in part because "the good life" has been equated with fast economic growth.*
>
> —*Danny Graham*
> *CEO*
> *Engage Nova Scotia*
> *Canada*

In New Zealand, the Indigenous Māori people's perspective of well-being prioritizes knowing one's ancestry, exercising rights to knowledge, and expressing culture through acts such as recounting traditional narratives. After engaging people from the Māori tribes and other groups, New Zealand included cultural identity as a well-being domain in its Living Standards Framework.

For Australia's Indigenous peoples, a well-being approach would show that advancing economic benefits alone isn't enough. A meaningful life focuses on "the relationship between Mother Earth, our homeland, and ourselves, our kin, our future, and our ancestors," says Bellagio participant Romlie Mokak, CEO at the Lowitja Institute in Australia. "If the denial of our cultures and our identities results in us only enjoying the same economic outcomes of others, that's completely suboptimal, because we'll lose ourselves as Indigenous peoples to get there," he says.

In the warlike conditions of Palestine, on the other hand, Giacaman and colleagues are developing new indicators related to suffering, such as humiliation, human insecurity, and deprivation. These critical measures of ill-being can make the often "invisible wounds" of trauma, isolation, conflict, and displacement visible, informing new programs and practices that support people to persist and endure. This radically different approach to well-being can be created only by engaging people to understand what matters to them in their unique situation.

Bellagio participants shared these examples, among others, of how a well-being lens can identify culturally-specific priorities and needs—as well as inequities and injustices—that can be masked by other indicators. This expanded definition of what matters can inform new approaches and create accountability for governments, businesses, and other actors.

This definition can only be created, however, through deep engagement of the grass roots. Listening to people and building trusting relationships with them is key in the iterative and dynamic grassroots engagement process, said multiple conference participants.

From the lens of our own experiences we can identify clearly the key drivers of change and priorities for our actions at a community and a national level.
—*José Molinas Vega*
Minister-Secretary of Planning for
Economic and Social Development
Republic of Paraguay

Confronting the roots of inequity: racism, colonialism, and protection of the status quo

In many parts of the world, inequities are caused by racism, colonialism, gender bias, and other forms of marginalization, which perpetuate structures, systemic inequities, cultural expectations, and narratives that protect and justify the status quo. Part of that status quo is a dominant narrative of economic growth, wealth, and consumption as the ultimate indicators of progress, which tacitly accepts a level of inequity as a norm. This, in turn, has shaped mindsets and behaviors and led to policies and systems that support economic inequality and the denial of basic human rights. Communities of color, Indigenous communities, and others subjected to persistent racism are denied voice and power, creating a generational cycle of oppression that impedes both current and future well-being.

The status quo is the problem. It's not just an economic argument.
—*Jennifer Prah Ruger*
Amartya Sen Professor of Health Equity, Economics, and Policy
University of Pennsylvania
United States

A focus on well-being has the potential to disrupt this status quo and to build currency for more equitable indicators of progress, shifting the narrative in powerful ways and driving changes in actions, policies, and practices that address inequity.

"Equity should be considered as a meta-indicator for all dimensions of well-being," says Éloi Laurent, senior economist at the Sciences Po Centre for Economic Research in France. Laurent stressed the need for disaggregated data that expose inequities along gender, racial, age, socioeconomic, and other dimensions to be useful and accurate for policy. "The way we choose to see, measure, and value these inequities (as opposed to the ones that remain invisible) depends on normative judgments and priorities that should be explicit."

Well-being data and concepts, designed in a collaborative way with communities, can show how inequities thwart progress, setting the stage for new narratives, policies, and other actions that advance both the well-being framework and equity.

Shifting power

The lens of well-being brings problems into focus, provides early warning signs of conditions that can spiral into crises, and clearly shows how groups do not share equally in access to prosperity and in positions of power. These are the "stories that the standard numbers often do not tell," as Bellagio participant Carol Graham, Leo Pasvolsky senior fellow at the Brookings Institution, and a professor at the University of Maryland, discusses extensively in chapter 3.

A well-being approach also clarifies power distribution, identifying groups that lack both representation and the full inclusion and power that make representation meaningful. For example, the aboriginal and Indigenous peoples of the world—making up about 370 million people in more than 70 countries—need a "voice with teeth," says Bellagio participant Walter Flores, executive director of the Center for the Study of Equity and Governance in Health Systems, based in Guatemala and working globally.

> *We can't advance a global agenda of well-being if we ignore 370 million Indigenous people that think differently than we think.*
>
> —*Walter Flores*
> *Executive Director*
> *Center for the Study of Equity and Governance in Health Systems*
> *Guatemala*

As an illustration of how lack of inclusion and power among Indigenous peoples leads to exclusionary policies that harm well-being, Flores says, "You cannot experience well-being unless your territory and the environment are being protected, because your survival depends on that." In Latin America, for example, Indigenous peoples told the government that they do not want destructive industries in their territories, citing the record of pollution in rivers and lakes. This can set up a clash between the quest for economic growth and the needs of the people. A well-being approach can encourage governments to listen to these groups, respect and act upon their preferences, and, ultimately, to shift power dynamics to include their voices in leadership and decision-making.

Fostering collaboration

A well-being approach can bring together people in fields such as health, economics, housing, education, and environmental protection, and can link the private and public sectors. "The well-being message and the well-being program are widely supported by lots of different groups in society," says Bellagio participant Tim Ng, deputy secretary and chief economic adviser of The New Zealand Treasury. As a commonly accepted framework for measuring progress, well-being brings diverse partners to the table and can lead to the development of equitable practices, programs, and policies that enable all people to lead the best lives possible. In Nova Scotia, for example, people from environmental groups, industry, anti-poverty groups, sports, academia, government, and community groups are working together to enhance the province's well-being framework.

By creating space for collaboration and alignment—a space where everyone can see themselves and their contributions—a well-being approach creates an opportunity for far more efficiency and impact. This includes the opportunity to link networks, social movements, agendas, financial and investment models, and other efforts, and a safe space to experiment. Benefits include encouraging open deliberation by governments and public participation in policymaking, deeply engaging grassroots organizations, and identifying opportunities for change.

Linking well-being of people and the environment, symbiotically

A segment of emerging well-being measurement, particularly in Western cultures, tends to be anthro-centric, looking first and foremost at the human condition. But for eternity, many Indigenous communities and environmentally focused cultures have taken an eco-centric approach, tightly connecting human well-being to environmental sustainability and the intrinsic value of the land to a culture or community.

Bellagio participants discussed the ways that well-being approaches, with their more holistic view of progress, can seamlessly link human and environmental conditions more effectively than other models. For the Indigenous peoples of Australia, Latin America, New Zealand, and North America, human well-being is inextricably linked with environmental sustainability and the intrinsic value of the land to the community. In Bhutan, a key component of the well-being approach is the interdependence of people and the natural world in the web of life, a perspective that has led to landmark environmental protection policies and resulted in Bhutan being the first carbon-negative nation.

As a result of climate change and other environmental crises, more attention is being given to the intersections of environmental and human health, the disparities of environmental justice, and the opportunities created by approaches that sustain health, life, and resources. Bellagio participant Laurent wrote about this connection in a paper he prepared for the Bellagio gathering: "Inequality increases the need for environmentally harmful and socially unnecessary economic growth, increases the ecological irresponsibility of the richest, diminishes the resilience of communities and societies, and weakens their collective ability to adapt to accelerating environmental change. It reduces the ability to offset the potential socially-regressive effects of environmental policies."

Creating a new expectation, demand, and accountability for well-being

As countries and cities prioritize well-being thinking and take different actions, individual and collective consciousness shifts toward the well-being of people, communities, and the planet. Consciousness shifts from a priority on economies that grow whether people thrive, to a priority on creating equitable and sustainable conditions for people to thrive that does not depend solely upon economic growth. Rather than being pulled by immediate and short-term gains, the compass will be guided by an intergenerational approach that plans for the future.

The way that people interpret data and conditions and develop solutions is likely to change under this new consciousness. "Me-first" behaviors, such as amassing tremendous personal wealth or making choices about natural resources that deplete the environment, will become less appealing as a well-being consciousness takes hold. Measures and definitions of progress will better align incentives with collective benefit, such as funding strong education systems and planning growth in ways that facilitate global sustainability and equity.

Bellagio participant Claire Nelson, lead futurist of the Futures Forum in the United States and the Caribbean, imagined life in 2030 under a well-being framework. "There's been a positive shift in our consciousness of who we are as humans to something that's global, planetary, and collective," she envisioned. If evolutionary, or eco-centric leadership and planetary consciousness were to become common ideas that people understood and took for granted, the use of resources to achieve a culture of well-being globally could be significantly improved, she says. A G-7-like organization focused on advancing well-being instead of economic growth could be established. Leaders in global organizations, such as the World Bank and the United Nations, could be trained, and future leaders could be groomed to work for the benefit of human and planetary well-being rather than personal gain.

> *Let's throw out some of the old ideas of what leadership looks like and teach them what it means to be a leader in a global planetary society.*
> —Claire A. Nelson
> *Lead Futurist*
> *The Futures Forum*
> *United States and the Caribbean*

With this shift in consciousness and expectation comes a collective challenge to historic assumptions and systems, and the tipping point to a focus on a well-being approach. "Very few radical shifts in society have taken place because of measurement or because we had data. It has usually required a social movement and people organizing in order to shift power," says Bellagio participant Mallika Dutt, founder and director of the global initiative Inter-Connected.

> *The most important task is to build the constituency that will be demanding and putting pressure on the authorities about a well-being agenda.*
> *—Walter Flores*
> *Executive Director*
> *Center for the Study of Equity and Governance in Health Systems*
> *Guatemala*

Nelson noted the power of the grass roots as a force in creating a well-being culture. It takes just 10 percent of a population to be committed to an idea for that idea to spread, according to a study by researchers at Rensselaer Polytechnic Institute.[1] This means that about 700 million of the world's 7 billion people would need to be committed to well-being. With about 370 million Aboriginal/Indigenous people who already believe in well-being, Nelson reasoned, that's about half of the people needed to create change. "So now it doesn't seem so impossible," she said.

Grassroots engagement is vital in both defining meaningful indicators and building community expectations for implementing a national well-being approach. If that engagement has been built, then "Once a country is ready to consider well-being indicators, a lot of the work will have already been done, and a lot of the politicians and others will already be on board," says Julia Kim, program director of the GNH Centre Bhutan, and Bellagio participant.

Focusing on the future and intergenerational leadership

"We're trying to create an elbow in the road that is fundamentally different from what had been before," says Bellagio participant Danny Graham, CEO at Engage Nova Scotia. "We're in the very early days of that elbow in the road. And in 50 years' time, it's probably still going to be very early in the days, given the size and complexity of this work." Bhutan, for example, first implemented its well-being approach in the 1970s and continues to refine and expand its application today, adapting to shifting realities and needs of its population in a global society. Well-being is not an end point, a destination to reach and declare victory. It evolves and emerges as "what matters most" changes, always with an eye toward the future.

A well-being approach facilitates this kind of long-term agenda setting. The New Zealand Treasury's well-being framework is a good example of this. Introduced in 2011, the Living Standards Framework informs policy development and resource allocation across the government. The Treasury's 2014 statement on the fiscal position for the next 40 years included future well-being challenges and considerations. The New Zealand government's 2019 well-being budget was designed to address the needs of both current and future generations.

> *If you are serious about future generations, then you need to recognize the tradeoff between drawing down capital to fund initiatives for the current population at the expense of future populations.*
>
> —*Tim Ng*
> *Deputy Secretary and Chief Economic Adviser*
> *The New Zealand Treasury*

To be truly future-oriented, a well-being approach must commit to intergenerational leadership, both to inform policies that will affect today's young people now and in the future, and to prepare future leaders to stay the course. Young people in their teens and twenties must be part of determining what matters most and developing and implementing well-being measures and actions, working alongside wise elders and experienced practitioners to question the status quo and existing assumptions.

Well-being initiatives around the world are focusing on engaging youth and intergenerational leadership. In Singapore, the Ministry of Health and two major universities are collaborating on a national initiative to develop future leaders who will adopt a "health and wealth" mindset over the dominant "wealth-first" mindset. Schools in Bhutan have a Gross National Happiness (GNH) curriculum to help young people understand GNH and to counteract increased exposure to a materialist culture through social media. Initiatives like these are "creating a new generation of people with a different value system," says Bellagio participant Kee-Seng Chia, founding dean of the National University of Singapore's School of Public Health.

The Path Ahead and the Vital Need to Ensure Equity

While participants agreed that a well-being approach can, and in many cases already does, provide many benefits and positive outcomes, we must "be careful to think about the enabling conditions for well-being in the local context," says

Kim. Key among these are truth telling about history and experiences, and ensuring that benefits are equitably shared.

Truth telling is essential

A well-being approach must address underlying causes of inequity, including systemic and structural racism. Truth telling is an important first step in the process. Only by revealing the truth of history, experience, and impact can there be healing and creation of a different future together. Blocking the truth cuts off power, as seen worldwide in the inaccurate and detrimental anti-migration narrative that continues to gain ground. Inequities due to racism have gotten far too little attention. "Since nobody wants to talk about racism, can we, as a proxy, use well-being as a variable in the Americas?" asks Nelson.

> *Communities of color historically continue to be on the short end of the stick with respect to structural oppression.*
>
> —*Anita Chandra*
> *Vice President and Director*
> *RAND Social and Economic Well-Being*
> *RAND Corporation*
> *United States*

Truth telling also involves reconciling cultural narratives and policies that have been unfavorable to some groups of people for many generations. For example, the Aboriginal and Torres Strait Islander people in Australia, whose cultures have existed for more than 60,000 years, have been living under colonization since the 1770s. According to Mokak, Australian governments try to steer the aboriginal people toward a Western lifestyle, ignoring their right to self-determination and their well-being directly connected to environmental sustainability. "There's very little trust between governments and Indigenous peoples," says Mokak.

> *Those who have arrived on our lands are not willing to own up to the truth of the history of the country.*
>
> —*Romlie Mokak*
> *CEO*
> *Lowitja Institute*
> *Australia*

Well-being's potential to illuminate and address inequities

"We have plenty of evidence showing that with new policies, the better-off benefit. It takes years for the worse-off to benefit from a new policy," says Flores. Carol Graham makes the argument that focusing on well-being may help mitigate this. While increases in average income often reduce the well-being of those below the average, she says, higher levels of average well-being tend to increase total well-being for all.

Still, great care is needed to ensure that well-being measures, policies, and actions are created collectively, with many voices and an inclusive power structure. Measures, policies, and actions must also be designed to illuminate and address inequities. They must reflect what matters most to people and communities, and not be another top-down approach. "We must ensure that one person's well-being doesn't supplant the well-being of others within the society," says Bellagio participant Richard E. Besser, president and CEO of the Robert Wood Johnson Foundation.

Conclusion: Well-Being Is an Imperative Now

"The well-being agenda isn't one that we've invented in different places. It is deeply embedded in the wisdom and traditions of people and in the lived experiences, aspirations, hopes, and values of people all over the world," says Dutt.

There is growing interest in the well-being approach as a way to define progress and to drive policies and practices based on what matters most to people and communities. Significant progress has been made in well-being measurement and its application to improve lives. International bodies have refined indicators and global commissions have advocated for including well-being in measures of progress. Some cities and countries are beginning to use well-being indicators to set policy and measure progress. "This is the moment to use the huge body of evidence on well-being and why things like equity matter," says Carol Graham.

And there is increasing urgency for a shift. In this time of great human conflict, displacement, and deaths of despair, there is a tremendous need for improved well-being. Economic indicators alone have failed to quantify and address increases in inequity, grave disparities in lived experiences, unsustainable draws on natural capital, and serious damage to intergenerational prosperity. Mounting measures of despair, and the nearly unprecedented levels of global migration due to violence and environmental change, demand a change in approach and an urgency for action.

Taking a well-being approach has the potential to inform choices that address inequity; improve the health and vitality of people, communities, and planet; and increase intergenerational equity. The time to move from measuring well-being to taking actions to improve well-being is now. "Could well-being be that creative emergent space for us to build the world that we all hold in our hearts differently than the structures that have gone before?" asked Dutt.

DEFINING WELL-BEING
AND INDICATORS
OF PROGRESS

Section 1 details the benefits of broadening the definition of progress to include well-being, and the rest of this book explores how to do that. First, though, a word about the well-being measures that help decision-makers both design and evaluate their approach.

Measures and indicators can inform and justify choices, help frame and advance agendas, and evaluate the effectiveness of actions. They can also influence narratives about what matters and shape ongoing decision-making and social consciousness. It's a self-fulfilling cycle: Societies count what they value, and place value on what gets counted.

For most of recent history, economic indicators (e.g., gross domestic product, housing starts, the consumer price index, unemployment rates, investment rates) have been used to assess progress. But as discussed in the preceding chapters, these types of measures often can mask inequity, miss early indicators for emerging threats, and fail to highlight non-economic assets and opportunities. In response to this shortcoming, new measures of well-being are gaining currency—not as an either-or alternative to economic measures but as a means of providing a complementary and more holistic set of indicators to better define progress and inform future-oriented goal setting and planning. As global interest and focus on well-being grow, how to best measure it is often at the center of exploration, discussion, and early action.

Well-being measures draw on psychology, neuroscience, anthropology, sociology, public health, economics, and many other disciplines to understand human flourishing and prosperity. Most of these measures include a combination of objective well-being (quantifiable indications of conditions), subjective well-being (self-reported life satisfaction measures), and the state of the environment and its impact on well-being. The blend of measures is crucial; relying on subjective measures alone can mask inequities, allow individual blame, and be manipulated to justify political agendas. Objective measures alone, on the other hand, can mask cultural context and ignore the wisdom of lived experience.

While the discourse at Bellagio focused on moving beyond measurement to action, the group emphasized the importance of getting the measures right and continuing to fine-tune indicators, as well as their application, to advance equity. Practitioners in the group emphasized that measures need to be simple and relevant to everyday people, but not overly simplistic or reduced to one number that masks context and nuance. Case studies illustrated how good data—readily understandable and culturally resonant—can become one of the drivers for policy and practice, and can help shape a new narrative that centers well-being as a key marker of progress. The researchers in the group discussed the evolution of measures and their use as a conceptual frame to drive change.

This section includes chapter 3, "The Stories the Numbers Do Not Tell: Measuring and Monitoring Well-Being in a Culture of Health," in which Bellagio participant Carol Graham, Leo Pasvolsky senior fellow at the Brookings Institution, and a professor at the University of Maryland, describes how well-being is measured, the associated strengths and weaknesses, and the opportunities to continue advancing well-being measurement. These ideas are further explored through the perspectives of the Bellagio participants in chapter 4, "Why the Dials on the Dashboard Matter: Discussion and Case Studies From Bellagio," which looks at the state of well-being measurement and discusses ways to make measures more meaningful. It also explores how measurement, while certainly not the impetus for every well-being approach, can be used as a lever for change.

As important and absorbing as refining the measures can be, the work must quickly shift beyond measurement science to application, action, and impact. It remains essential to measure and analyze how taking a well-being approach shifts policy, practice, and culture in order to determine what works, and document impact. As one participant noted: "We can have perfect measures and go nowhere."

The Stories the Numbers Do Not Tell

Measuring and Monitoring Well-Being in a Culture of Health

CAROL GRAHAM, AB, MA, DPHIL

Leo Pasvolsky Senior Fellow, the Brookings Institution, United States
College Park Professor, the University of Maryland, United States

Building a Culture of Health is a multifaceted challenge that, at minimum, requires ensuring that access to health care is available to all; more broadly, it entails addressing the social determinants of health—the economic and social conditions, from income to education to community context, that affect health risks and outcomes. We are far from that broader objective in many countries around the world. In the United States, for example, unprecedented prosperity coexists with deep desperation and rising premature mortality rates, inequality of incomes and opportunities, unequal access to health care, and large differences in happiness, hope, and stress across rich and poor. Conditions such as high economic growth, increasing labor market returns to the highly skilled, and rising life expectancy coexist with increasing numbers of prime-age workers with less than a college degree dropping out of the labor force and experiencing rising rates of deaths of despair and other markers of ill-health.[1]

The aggregate numbers and standard measures typically used to track progress—growth rates, unemployment figures, and stock market trends—mask this underlying crisis of social ill-being. In contrast, well-being metrics uncover the stories that these numbers do not tell.

My own research, for example, found deep desperation among less-than-college-educated whites—juxtaposed against much higher levels of optimism among poor minorities—well before the data on rising premature mortality was discovered.[2-4] Since then we have established robust matches between the trends in ill-being—desperation, stress, and worry—and premature mortality at the individual level and across race and place. In our most recent research, based on longer-term data, we find that the drops in hope and optimism among the less than college educated began as early as the 1970s, roughly corresponding to the beginning of the decline of manufacturing jobs and other adverse indicators.[5]

Had we been tracking well-being regularly in the United States, as countries such as the United Kingdom already do, the metrics—and their inclusion in the political discourse and policymaking arenas—would have sounded the alarm bells about desperation and ill-being well before they manifested in mortality rates. A focus on individual and community-level well-being might well have resulted in a very different trajectory. We can and should use these metrics systematically as a means to monitor the well-being of our society, and more generally as a complement to standard income and health indicators to provide a more comprehensive and realistic compass for decision-making.

As complementary measures of progress, well-being metrics have the power to influence the public narrative. By illuminating how standard income-based metrics alone can pick up the wrong story, well-being metrics create an opportunity for public discussion of the state of society, including how many of the things that matter are missing in the standard metrics. This new narrative, in turn, has the potential to redefine how we assess "success" and pursue progress, a shift that ultimately affects mindsets, attitudes, social norms, and decisions.

A narrative based on broadly shared well-being has the potential to reduce many political and policy divides, and contributes to building a shared Culture of Health. This is in part because well-being, unlike income or political resources, which are both finite and unequally shared, has an indivisible quality with positive externalities across individuals and places. Higher average incomes at the country or city level often reduce the well-being of those below the average, due to comparison effects.[6] In contrast, higher levels of average well-being tend to *increase* total well-being, regardless of where people are in the well-being distribution. There are rarely winners and losers, and more well-being at the individual level typically translates into more well-being at the community level. Well-being has a positive relationship with many health outcomes, meanwhile, and the lessons are generalizable across individuals and communities.[7]

One of the most compelling things about these metrics is that the average person identifies more closely and naturally with them than with standard income-based data. For example, endless messages about smoking being bad for health often fall on deaf ears. Yet the message that people who smoke are less happy than those who do not smoke tends to get much more attention. Knowledge about the well-being of one's own community, meanwhile, tends to have more impact than do anonymous national indicators. Involving people with lived experience in the communities in the implementation and/or dissemination of results tends to lead to higher levels of involvement and action by the communities themselves.* That same involvement has its own well-being effects on those who participate, particularly in communities where respondents feel isolated and/or left behind.

Why Is It Time for a Well-Being Framework?

We have made much progress since the days when a majority of social scientists, and particularly economists, were extremely skeptical of research on happiness and well-being. In 20 years, the approach has gone from a nascent collaboration between a few psychologists and economists (myself included) to an accepted method in economics and in the social sciences more generally. What began as an experimental use of surveys of subjective well-being has become a robust measurement science that aims to understand the determinants of well-being beyond income alone. A range of countries and municipalities are now using well-being metrics to inform policy design, to monitor policy progress, and to assess policy outcomes, providing a wealth of experience to build upon.

The progress has been stunning for those of us involved early on. I participated in many steps along the way, including serving on a U.S. National Academy of Sciences panel that, in collaboration with the Behavioral Insights Team in the United Kingdom and with the OECD Better Life Initiative, sought to establish and disseminate the best measurement practices and applications.

Rapid take-up and usage of the metrics began in 2010. One reason for the increased receptivity to the approach may have been the global financial crisis, which shook faith in standard economic models and demonstrated that the many bubbles inflating housing, financial, and other markets were in the end deleterious to the welfare—and ultimately the health—of much of society. Regardless of the reasons, meanwhile, the moment is ripe with opportunities to use the metrics across a range of academic disciplines and public policy questions, with public health and its social determinants being a natural candidate.

---

* See, for example, the long list of interventions with positive outcomes based on the city of Santa Monica's well-being index and related local efforts (*https://designmattersatartcenter.org/proj/wellbeing-santa-monica*), as well as the many evaluations of such interventions in deprived communities by the What Works Well Being team in the United Kingdom (*www.whatworkswellbeing.org*).

Well-Being as an Aggregate Indicator of Progress?

Using well-being as an aggregate indicator of progress is a possibility, but it is important to tread cautiously in this area. Using the individual metrics, based on robust measures of well-being and implemented according to best practice, as indicators of progress (or lack thereof) has great potential to enhance our objective indicators of income and health. Indeed, the most important information that comes from using both subjective and objective indicators—a combination that is a hallmark of well-being metrics—comes from discrepancies in what the different indicators reveal.

Well-being metrics often uncover novel and surprising trends, patterns, paradoxes, and stories behind the standard numbers. As noted above, standard unemployment rates, for example, do not include individuals who have dropped out of the labor market—they simply drop out of the denominator. In the United States, low unemployment rates coexist with rising numbers—and desperation—of prime-age individuals who are out of the labor force, a number projected to reach 25 percent of prime-age males by 2025.[8] China experienced a slightly different progress paradox in the 1990s, in which unprecedented growth rates and movements out of poverty were accompanied by dramatic drops in life satisfaction and increases in suicide, which were most prevalent among the new high-income earners in the private sector.[9]

Well-being metrics uncover phenomena such as failure to report poor health because of poor norms and low expectations in many contexts. They can assess the negative effects of inequity on future expectations and related investments in the labor market and in health. At the same time, they also highlight unexpected optimism and resilience among deprived populations. Daily experience or "hedonic" metrics, meanwhile, are particularly well suited for assessing daily quality of life and the well-being effects of different health conditions, based on the responses of people who are actually experiencing them. By measuring affect and mood as recalled the day before, these metrics allow us to assess how individuals *actually experience* different working and living arrangements, different health conditions or care-giving arrangements, and a host of other activities ranging from commuting to work to spending time with friends and family.

A note of caution is necessary, however. Much of the debate on well-being—and in particular national happiness—as a progress indicator ends up in discussions of replacing gross domestic product (GDP) with Gross National Happiness (GNH). In my view, that idea is misguided. It dismisses standard indicators that are essential to measuring economic and health progress. That approach would also forfeit the capacity to explore what the discrepancies between objective and subjective indicators tell us. In addition, that sort of discussion typically ends up losing the attention and potential support of a wide range of actors—academics, policymakers, and politicians, for example—who are willing to use new indicators but not to toss out the baby (GDP) with the bath water. Unfortunately, that split plays into political divisions as well, with GNH typically viewed as a "left-wing" agenda, at least in places such as the United States. Finally, there is also political risk involved, as having governments in the business of *promoting* "happiness" rather than measuring and tracking the well-being of their populations opens the door to political manipulation of the metrics and the findings.

It is important to avoid these divisions and to provide a realistic narrative about well-being as a progress indicator. This requires emphasizing the measurement science and the nuances that underlie any aggregate measure, and making the distinct dimensions of well-being very clear. The users of these indicators—especially the public—need to be aware that any aggregate indices are based on large numbers of individual responses that yield discrete findings across people, places, and races. The disaggregated data provide a more robust toolkit as inputs into policy discussions and assessments. Aggregate well-being indicators can serve as warning lights on a dashboard: they point either to vulnerabilities in particular places or cohorts, to positive trends that provide broader lessons, or to both. As such, in my view, we should consider having traditional GDP and aggregate well-being indicators on the same policymaking dashboard, reported in the media, and included in policymaking debates.

Best Practice in Measurement and in Practice

Clarity on measurement—and, in particular, making it clear that the research does not involve asking individuals what makes them happy—is essential for best measurement practice *and* for avoiding political manipulation of the measures. If it is clear to the public that the measures are part of normal statistics collection and not tagged to specific governments or political issues, the measures become more difficult to politicize or manipulate. As noted above, if particular governments proclaim happiness to be an objective of policy as a political strategy, or establish departments designed to *promote* happiness, the metrics themselves can become suspect. In contrast, incorporating the metrics into particular processes—as in the case of New Zealand's well-being budgeting, discussed in chapter 9—is a much more effective way of incorporating them into policy.

Clarity in communication of the results is also important. To create an effective and credible narrative, public messages should be as simple as possible and quite clear on what we can and cannot measure. They should also be tailored to specific populations. While some findings—such as the average effects of income, employment, and health—are generic to well-being among most populations, many others vary across individuals and groups. As such, it is important to have well-being in the mix of mainstream policy indicators, while not being an exclusive indicator. Well-being indicators are most effective when used in the broader context of many other (complementary) objectives of policy, which typically use standard income measures or health indicators as an initial benchmark. The most novel insights, meanwhile, typically come from the instances when there are gaps in the findings that come from different metrics, for example, when well-being metrics tell us one story and GDP tells another. We need both.

Surveys are a standard data collection mechanism for well-being data, and there is now established best practice for implementing well-being surveys. A key consensus is on the importance of measuring *three distinct dimensions of well-being*—hedonic, evaluative, and eudaimonic—to paint a complete picture.[10]

- **Hedonic metrics** capture individuals' moods and affective states as they go through their daily activities. Hedonic metrics are most applicable for measuring quality of daily lives. One useful application, for example, is evaluating the short-term effects of various health conditions and their treatments as an input into choice of care decisions.
- **Evaluative metrics** capture individuals' evaluations of their lives as a whole. These metrics are best for assessing life satisfaction and other aspects of life course well-being. This includes respondents' agency to choose the kinds of lives they want to lead.
- **Eudaimonic metrics** are the newest. They capture the Aristotelian concept of well-being, which combines having sufficient means (the Greek "eu") with having control over one's destiny ("daimon"). These metrics ask individuals if they have purpose or meaning in their lives (for an example of the kinds of findings that come from the metrics that assess this dimension, see Graham and Nikolova, 2015).[11]

Ideal measurement practice includes all three sets of measures, as they each reveal different elements of quality of life and well-being, ranging from daily moods to life course evaluations to purposefulness or lack thereof.

My research on very poor populations around the world and, more recently, among deprived or downwardly mobile cohorts in the United States, demonstrates the comprehensive story these three dimensions, taken together, reveal. Many lives are overwhelmed by negative hedonic experiences, such as stress that is due to circumstances beyond their control.[12,13] While these same individuals may express that they are happy in a daily sense, either due to positive character traits or to adaptive expectations, they tend to score much lower on life evaluations. This is not a surprise, as they have much less agency or capacity to plan for and invest in their futures. Individuals with more means tend to score higher on life evaluations, and while they may experience stress, it is more likely to be associated with goal achievement rather than with constant negative shocks. Eudaimonic metrics, meanwhile, often find differences between experiences that are purposeful but not pleasurable, such as reading the same story to a small child for the fifteenth time, and pleasurable but not purposeful, such as watching television.

It is important to measure positive and negative hedonic experiences separately. Smiling and stress, for example, capture distinct emotions that are not the analogues of each other. Life evaluations, in contrast, capture the same cognitive assessment on a continuous scale. Measurement of all of the questions, meanwhile, should be on unipolar scales going from low to high, such as from not at all happy to very happy or not stressed to very stressed. Bi-polar scales with responses running in different directions, such as dissatisfied versus very satisfied, tend to result in skewed distributions. Life evaluations in particular, meanwhile, should appear upfront in the surveys, so that preceding questions, such as about individuals' jobs, incomes, or marriages, do not bias the responses. Finally, there are day-of-the-week effects, with Sunday typically being the day with the highest life satisfaction levels, and Monday the lowest. Adjusting for day-of-the-week effects is important to accurate measurement.

Perhaps the most important measurement and implementation clarification is that the approach is not asking respondents if particular things (e.g., income) or activities (e.g., smoking or exercising) make them happy or stressed. Respondents are not aware that we are linking the latter set of questions with their well-being reports, as that would introduce bias. Surveys begin with respondents' reported well-being along the dimensions noted above, and then collect extensive information on respondents' socioeconomic and demographic traits.*

Once these data are collected, we control for the variables that have stable patterns across individuals, countries, and time, such as age, income, marital and employment status, and health. See **Figure 1** on page 36. We can then explore the well-being associations of variables that vary more across people and populations, such as commuting time, smoking and other health behaviors, as

---

* We analyze the data via econometric equations taking the following form: $W_{it} = a + \beta x_{it} + \varepsilon_{it}$ in which W_{it} is the reported well-being (hedonic, evaluative, or eudaimonic) of individual i at time t, and βx_{it} is a vector of individual traits such as age, income, gender, employment status, marital status, objective or reported health, area of residence, and so forth. The epsilon/error term captures innate individual traits that we are unable to observe.

well as macroeconomic and institutional arrangements, such as inflation and un-employment rates, inequity, and governance quality, among many others.*[14-16]

Figure 1. Gallup World Poll 2010–2017: Determinants of life satisfaction around the world[1]

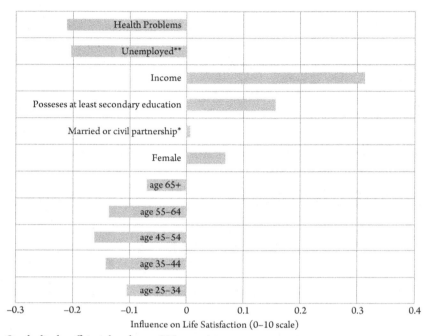

Influence on Life Satisfaction (0–10 scale)

Standardized coefficients based on an OLS regression.
* "Married or Civil Partnership" is compared to the "Single" marital status category.
** "Unemployed" is compared to the "Employed for an Employer" employment category.

Examples of Best Practice Implementation

There are numerous examples of the usage of well-being metrics to assess, mon-itor, and improve well-being at the community, city, and national levels.

- The city of Santa Monica constructed a citywide, multi-dimensional well-being index in 2013 and has used the results from that index to undertake

---

* In addition, because much of well-being is innately determined, the error term actually includes important information. Some research (including my own) attempts to use this information as a proxy for innate character traits and to explore the associations of those traits with individuals' outcomes in the labor, health, and social arenas. This research is strongly suggestive of a channel of causality running from well-being to better outcomes in the future. It is distinct from the research that attempts to tease out the determinants of life satisfaction and other dimensions of well-being and is becoming an entirely new area of exploration in both economics and the biological sciences.

multiple projects to enhance community and city-level well-being.*[17] (See the afterword by Julia Rusk, former chief of civic wellbeing for the city of Santa Monica, for more information.)

- The What Works Wellbeing (WWWB)[†] initiative in the United Kingdom provides low-cost interventions, such as access to the arts or incentives for new forms of commuting to work (e.g., better public transport or bike lanes). WWWB then has academics use well-being metrics to assess the effects of these interventions and disseminate the results both to the communities and more broadly.[18]

- The U.K. Office of National Statistics, meanwhile, now includes four well-being questions (life satisfaction, happy yesterday, anxious yesterday, and purpose/meaning in life—the so-called ONS4) in its annual statistics collection.[19] As a result, British citizens are regularly able to see how well-being has changed across population cohorts, districts, and time. Policymakers also are able to use these data to identify vulnerable populations and places. The measures initially were not understood by the public and became the subject of some political criticism. However, because they were collected using best practice and as part of a normal annual statistics gathering exercise, they have now become part of the normal policy discourse and media coverage.

Unanswered Questions

In addition to the now extensive knowledge about how a focus on well-being and the use of well-being metrics can contribute to better policy design and to monitoring and evaluation of policy progress, there are a number of unanswered questions. I focus here on questions that are relevant to the proposal to use well-being as a progress indicator.

- **Cardinality, ordinality,[‡] and public priorities.** The metrics use ordinal response categories that do not assume cardinality. Life satisfaction, for example, is assessed on a 0 to 11 scale. The patterns in the answers to this question tend to be consistent across people, places, and time. But we cannot assume, for example, that a score of 8 on the life satisfaction scale is equivalent to twice

---

* For example, see *https://designmattersatartcenter.org/proj/wellbeing-santa-monica*

† For more information, see *www.whatworkswellbeing.org*

‡ Cardinal measures assume that the numbers on the responses have an actual value, so 4 is twice the value of 2. Yet ordinal measures are simply scaled categories that respondents place themselves in, but without the underlying assumption that category 4 has a value that is twice that of category 2. In reality, though, the measures operate in a similar fashion.

as much life satisfaction as a scale of 4 (although in reality they mirror cardinality in econometric equations). For policy purposes, though, we must attach weights if the metrics are going to be useful in policy. Should we prioritize those respondents in misery (such as those below 4 on the scale)? Do we worry about raising the life satisfaction for those near the top of the scale? Do we reduce misery or enhance aggregate well-being? These are distinct objectives, and determining the relative weights will require public as well as academic discussion and, in a way, mirror the debates over targeted versus universal social welfare policies.

- **Scale interpretation.** Another question that stands out is how the public can or should interpret the scales. If we tell an uninformed layperson that national average happiness increased from 6.2 to 6.9 in the past year, that person would not know if that was good, bad, or indifferent, even though scholars would know it was significant. If metrics are to be included in policy, more work is necessary to explain the magnitude of score changes to the public. There will be a natural learning process as the metrics become more common in the public domain. Today, the average person on the street knows that a 1 percent increase in the unemployment rate is a bad thing, and that a 0.1 percent increase is not significant. The same person would likely have no idea how many people those numbers entail (indeed the answer is not that many, as these are percentages of the unemployed pool). The public reaction to movements in the Dow Jones index is similar: While most people do not know what the actual numerical change represents (or how the index is constructed), they understand what order of magnitude signals a significant change in the markets. Yet, as the figures appear so often in the media and in public discourse, the public knows roughly what they mean. The same would occur if well-being metrics were routinely reported.

- **Adaptation: The Happy Peasant and Frustrated Achiever Problem.** A more difficult question, meanwhile, is that of adaptation. It is well known (and I have written about this extensively[20]) that people are remarkably adaptable to many experiences (good and bad), and can return to their natural level of well-being. That creates a challenge for the metrics. For example, if a very poor person in bad health says that they are quite happy or satisfied with their health, do we know whether that is true or whether they have learned to live with bad conditions that they have no expectations of surmounting? If the latter, then the responses and the metrics based upon them could be very misleading about actual well-being. We are able to get around this in two ways. The first is an area of small but growing research on what people do and do not adapt to, which provides some markers. The second is the use of vignettes and other survey methods to test differences in how people of different cultures, races, gender, and income levels answer well-being questions, which in turn allows for scale adjustment. Meanwhile, better understanding of why people adapt and to what would provide important insights into the determinants of human well-being. This raises the question of what we cannot fully measure. While there are consistent patterns in the determinants of well-being worldwide, and the vignette approaches provide insights into different cultural perspectives on well-being and how people experience it, there are surely aspects of these differences that we are not able to capture precisely.

How Subjective Well-Being Metrics Can Contribute to New Efforts to Enhance Resilience and Well-Being Going Forward

My research on inequity in well-being and deaths of despair highlights a crisis of ill-being in the United States that merits our attention and alarm. Yet there are also surprising levels of hope and optimism among some groups experiencing objective challenges, which in turn suggest major differences in resilience across races and places. Better understanding of these differences in resilience will be an important facet of the solution to this crisis. A key question is whether individuals can learn to be more resilient. If so, are the lessons tangible enough to incorporate into well-being-based policy? While I cannot answer these questions fully at this point, some examples of work in the field indicate emerging strategies.

- One example, from my latest research and collaboration at the community level, is the Maryland Behavioral Health Association's Division of Child and Adolescent Mental Health, which is working with children of all ages to expose them to strategies that enhance resilience. This is particularly important for children living with high levels of trauma, for example, children as young as 3 or 4 years old whose parents have substance addictions, and who come to school in a state of stress. The MBHA's strategies include enhancing a sense of competency, caring, and respect for self and others; problem-solving and coping skills; and optimism and hope for the future. They also aim to help children reframe stress and to help seek purpose and meaning. While this is largely uncharted territory, the effort has already yielded tangible results and lessons for other communities. The basic proposition is that resilience is something we can teach and foster. *Well-being metrics can serve as design and assessment tools in this process.**

- Another example is the work of Diana Yazzie Devine and others from Native American Connections, who work with patients with opioid use disorder and their families in Native American communities.[21] A common theme running through the success stories in these programs, as well as others I have learned about, is the importance of having a connection that allows individuals in distress to seek help as part of building resilience. That connection can be a family member, a friend, or a member of the community—the human connection seems to matter more than what the relationship is. My research on desperation among white people living in poverty in rural and suburban areas highlights the lack of such connections as a key factor that defines the most desperate places and people. *Again, well-being metrics can serve as useful diagnostic tools, such as in detecting stress and desperation, and to evaluate the effectiveness of interventions.*

- Another example comes from my experimental research on the determinants of resilience among adolescents living on low incomes in Peru, which includes a detailed 400-person survey of 18- to 19-year-olds in a large poor and near-poor urban district of Lima. A remarkable 85 percent of the respondents aspire to completing college or postgraduate education. In response to a follow-up question, 95 percent of those respondents report that they can indeed achieve that objective. Not one of these adolescents has a parent who has completed college, and almost all of those with high aspiration have experienced one or more negative shocks in the past, including a parent leaving the household, the illness or death of a family member, or having experienced a crime or robbery. On the one hand, these adolescents have learned to cope and have learned resilience. Yet there is clearly a role for family and community in fostering that resilience. This is something that we will explore in detail in a repeat survey, in which we will also explore whether hope and resilience indeed actually lead to better future outcomes for these adolescents.[22] *Well-being metrics were foundational in the study design and in helping to understand the role of hope.*

- As a final, upcoming example, we are hoping to field the resilience survey in neighboring poor black and white communities in Missouri. We hope this will complement and deepen our previous work on the geography of desperation in the United States, work that empirically highlights the importance of culture and community in fostering optimism and hope among different

---

* Indeed, I am working with the MBHA to incorporate the metrics into several of their resilience building programs.

groups.[23] *Well-being metrics once again can tell us stories that the traditional numbers fail to capture.*

Collecting the common lessons that emerge from this nascent body of community-level work on resilience can serve an important role in the broader strategy of building a culture of health *and* well-being.

Conclusion

We now have a developed measurement science, growing consensus on best practice, and increased acceptance of the approach—and the importance—of well-being among many academics and policymakers around the world. We also have many national, local, and community-level initiatives that provide insights into what works, as well as what does not. Measurement is vital, and we must keep using and fine-tuning it as a tool to both better assess and understand human well-being and how people are doing, and to change the established narrative about economic and social progress. It is also critical to better understanding the elements of human well-being that we do not yet know how to measure.

Incorporating measures of well-being to provide a more nuanced view of how people are doing, to inform policies to address serious pockets of ill-being and to enhance aggregate societal well-being, and to create a new narrative about social progress is a proposition whose time has come.

Why the Dials on the Dashboard Matter

Discussion and Case Studies From Bellagio

Measurement can be both a driver and a signpost of social change. It can tell us where we are and how far we still have to go, whether our direction is on course or off track, whether our engine of change is running smoothly or needs a tune-up, and what actions will help us reach the destination. In an inequitable world, measurement can help us see where the patterns and variations are, whether differences are shrinking or growing, and whether the differences are due to unfair but avoidable circumstances (inequity) or the uneven distribution of resources (inequality). In this way, measurement enables us to understand paradoxes in individual and societal progress so we can tell a more comprehensive and precise story. And measurement can be a powerful tool for shifting narratives about how things are going and about what matters.

Well-being measurement is not merely a single number or a set of indices, but also a conceptual frame to drive high-impact change. It enables us to expand the notion of health far beyond the absence of disease, to expand the definition of progress far beyond economic measures alone, and to support a policy agenda that is rooted in socio-political and cultural context.

When applied to a well-being framework, measurement and data analysis become more complicated and nuanced. Although measurement was not the major focus of the Bellagio gathering, and is certainly not the only starting point or driver of change in a well-being approach, it was a constant thread running through the conversations. In the group's exploration of shifting mindsets and narratives, informing an equitable approach, generating accurate data, and stimulating meaningful action by communities and policymakers, a clear theme emerged: Measurement plays an essential role in advancing well-being.

That said, the state of measurement is incomplete. Metrics and definitions must be further refined and expanded to include well-being measures as a complement to economic vitality and other indicators. This chapter pursues that theme with a brief look at the state of measurement, measurement's role in advancing both a well-being framework and actual well-being outcomes, what makes measures meaningful, how to interpret and use data to drive change, and next steps for measuring well-being.

The State of Well-Being Measurement

Governments, international bodies, and dominant public narratives have long defined progress in terms of economic health and growth. The chief indicator has been gross domestic product (GDP), which refers to the value of goods and services produced.[1]

The challenge is that GDP "counts" many things that have financial costs or value but do not contribute to well-being and may, in fact, diminish it, such as incarceration, oil spills, natural disasters, massive development, and cars and machines that gobble natural resources. Metrics like these tend to ignore or mask conditions that indicate well-being, such as life satisfaction, health and mental health, happiness, quality of life, a sense of autonomy, social connectedness, and the like.[2,3] By focusing the dashboard almost exclusively on economic indicators, measurement practices have failed to help us understand or make progress on other important conditions that affect well-being.

> Gross national product* . . . measures everything except that which makes life worthwhile. And it can tell us everything about America except why we are proud that we are Americans.
> —Robert F. Kennedy[4]

A shift is underway around the world to define and measure the conditions and outcomes of equitable well-being. From the World Health Organization (WHO) to the Organisation for Economic Co-operation and Development (OECD), economic and public health leaders are helping to promote an evidence-based understanding of human well-being. For example, OECD's Better Life Initiative publishes a regularly updated set of well-being indicators[5] that many countries use as a base and then augment or adapt to match local contexts. Its How's Life report measures current well-being for individuals and households, and across population groups, in the domains of material living conditions (e.g., income and wealth, jobs and earnings, housing conditions) and quality of life (e.g., health status, work-life balance, education and skills, social connections, civic

---

* Precursor to gross domestic product (GDP).

engagement and governance, environmental quality, personal security, and life satisfaction). The index also uses indicators of different types of capital to assess future (or sustained) well-being.[6]

Global commissions charged with refining measures of progress have advocated for the inclusion of well-being indicators. That is the case with the European Social Survey, for example, which is a biennial cross-national survey of attitudes and behavior established in 2001. It tracks indicators such as social trust, citizen involvement, economic morality, welfare attitudes, ageism, trust in justice, democracy, health inequalities, climate change and energy use, justice and fairness, and digital social contacts.[7] In addition, well-being metrics now are required as part of cost-benefit analyses that inform policies within several countries, and many municipalities are planning community development and vitality strategies around well-being goals. For example:

- In the **United Kingdom**, Happy City works with numerous municipalities to use measurement data to establish new narratives that "reset the compass" toward the well-being of people, places, and the planet. The Thriving Places Index, published for 373 local governance authorities, measures the local conditions needed for people to thrive, balanced with whether they are being delivered equitably and sustainably. Another measurement tool, the Happiness Pulse, measures how well people actually are doing in terms of emotional, behavioral, and relational well-being; it can be used with individuals, households, organizations, communities, and entire local authority areas.
- In **Canada**, data collected through the Canadian Index of Wellbeing will inform prototype projects to shift cultural narratives, illuminate the full cost of public policy decisions, and enhance factors such as community vitality, social integration, a sense of belonging, social trust, and strong relationships.
- In **Bhutan**, the Gross National Happiness (GNH) Index is based on a survey of thousands of Bhutanese living in every district in the country. Using data on 33 indicators across nine domains, analysts create a well-being profile for each survey respondent. The individual profiles are aggregated to create a national index; the index then can be analyzed by demographic characteristic and by GNH domain.[8,9] Policymakers use the GNH index to identify individuals and populations that need attention, consider the potential effects of proposed policies, and evaluate the effectiveness of interventions over time.[10]
- In **New Zealand**, the government published its first well-being budget in 2019. "We're embedding [a] notion of making decisions that aren't just about growth for growth's sake, but how our people are faring," New Zealand Prime Minister Jacinda Ardern said at the World Economic Forum's annual meeting in January 2019. "How [are] their overall well-being and their mental health?

How is our environment doing? These are the measures that will give us a true measure of our success."

Within this movement to incorporate measures of well-being is an effort to include reflections on the cultural dimensions that, as Bellagio participant Nils Fietje, research officer for the World Health Organization, says, "become explicit through literature, through art, through journalism, through a variety of forums where the concerns and worries and questions around well-being are given voice." This type of evidence is no less important, powerful, or meaningful than numerical data, Bellagio participants agreed.

New Zealand's Well-Being Framework and Measures Drive Policymaking

In 2018, the New Zealand Treasury released a fully-revised version of its Living Standards Framework and accompanying dashboard of indicators* to measure national well-being. The framework, which grew out of a seven-year design process, draws on international research, measurement work by OECD, and decades of public debate about what New Zealanders value. It features 12 domains of current well-being: income and wealth, housing, jobs, health, knowledge and skills, leisure, safety and security, environment, civic engagement and governance, social connection, life satisfaction, and cultural identity. It also considers how the well-being of future generations will be sustained or improved by tracking natural, physical/financial, social, and human capital, and the resilience of current and future well-being.

The Treasury is using the framework and dashboard, along with other economic and fiscal frameworks, to inform policy development and resource allocation across the government. Future work includes better processes to monitor and evaluate whether existing policies promote well-being. The government's policy agenda features five well-being priorities: aiding the transition to a sustainable and low-emissions economy; supporting a thriving nation in the digital age; lifting Māori and Pacific incomes, skills, and opportunities; reducing child poverty; and supporting mental health for all New Zealanders.[11]

See chapter 9 for a full discussion by Bellagio participant Tim Ng, deputy secretary and chief economic adviser of the New Zealand Treasury.

---

* For more information, see *www.treasury.govt.nz/lsfdashboard*.

Measurement's Role in Advancing Well-Being

Measurement has the potential to motivate and persuade people and institutions to act. Knowing exactly how well or unwell a population is, and what impact that has on society, can persuade individuals, communities, systems, businesses, philanthropists, civil-society organizations, and governments to take action. The data collected through measurement raise awareness about how specific communities are affected and suggest a path to remediation, whether through changes in policies and resource allocations, grassroots mobilizing, litigation, education, or other means. For example, after recognizing that early language skills are essential for proficient reading—and that a large proportion of 3- and 4-year-olds have oral language difficulties— New Zealand's government allocated funding in its Well-Being Budget for the Ministry of Education to give this population targeted support. Similarly, the country's Ministry of Justice received targeted funding to provide cognitive behavioral therapy, functional family therapy, and professional mentoring to 14- to 16-year-olds whose experiences put them at risk of committing criminal offenses.

To be certain, economic indicators and development remain an integral part of New Zealand's considerations, and the Bellagio group repeatedly emphasized that this is not about doing away with economic measures. "Some discomfort I was feeling during the [first day of dialogue] was about forgetting what economics and what the development of formal markets and capitalism has actually delivered, which is lifting hundreds of millions of people out of poverty," said Ng. "Some fundamental truths about lots of people in both developed and developing countries is that they just want a job, and they want higher incomes, and they want low child mortality, and they want a reduction in premature deaths through preventable causes and things like that. And these are things that economic development actually delivers."

Measurement galvanizes people to address well-being across political divides. Measures of well-being can provide a tangible and objective way to look at issues that in other settings could be perceived as partisan. For example, if the end goal is defined as the well-being of people and the planet, then planning decisions are taken out of short-term cycles and political polarities. As Bellagio participant Liz Zeidler, chief executive of Happy City in the United Kingdom, illustrates: "Should a new cultural center be in a big, out-of-town setting, paid for by global investors, or should it be co-funded by regional and national backers close to and involving the community it serves? On purely GDP-based, short-term metrics, out-of-town wins for its lower initial outlay, money spent on transporting people there, etc. But against well-being metrics we see its impact on the environment, air pollution, jobs, and profit all sucked out of the local community, lack of building community pride and belonging, lack of positive impact on local enterprises—this makes the decision easier to make in favor of people and [the] planet, not just profit."

Moreover, an inclusive and collaborative approach to developing measures can result in measures that are perceived as less partisan and are more meaningful to diverse interest groups and, therefore, more likely to motivate action.

Measurement helps capture and reflect on differences in well-being between populations, over time, and across places. While an economic report might paint a picture of unprecedented prosperity overall, looking at indicators through a well-being perspective will reveal that not everyone shares in the prosperity—and that, in some cases, even the most economically prosperous are not necessarily "well." Think of the data on vast disparities in income distribution captured by economist Thomas Piketty (discussed in chapter 6), for example, or the findings on rising rates of deaths of despair—suicides and drug overdoses prompted by tension, trauma, and ill-being—among white people in the United States.

Measurement can drive narratives and discourse about well-being. Narrative, like measurement, was a cross-cutting theme at Bellagio, and is discussed in-depth in section 3. Narratives are collections of stories that work together as a system[12] to convey an interpretation of the world and how it works.[13,14] They are reflected in cultural products,[15] such as language, art, news and entertainment media, and advertising and political messages. The repeated expression of specific narratives also plays a role in shaping culture.[16] Narratives can emerge organically, in response to the accumulation of similar stories developed through a social process, or they can be intentionally created and deployed as a tool for social change or oppression. Narratives that are based on the attitudes, beliefs, and values held by people in positions of power within a given culture, system, or social structure tend to become dominant narratives. These narratives reflect prevailing notions of who holds power and how they use it, while also creating and perpetuating the power dynamics.

Narratives are both a tool for and focus of social change: Efforts to shift dominant narratives challenge assumptions, advance a new view of reality and what is to be expected, and aim to shift power. Measurement and narrative have a symbiotic relationship when it comes to well-being: Measures of well-being can drive new narratives about progress, while narratives about what matters and what a society values can underscore the need for new metrics to capture well-being. For example, incorporating alternate indicators of well-being—such as the amount of time parents can spend with their children versus working; the level of social capital experienced by residents (e.g., community vitality, social integration, sense of belonging, social trust, strong relationships); the ability of older people to live in the community versus in an institution—creates an opportunity for discourse about what development (and over-development) means for society, what impact inequity has on well-being, and what might be gained rather than lost by pursuing greater equity. Bellagio participant Mallika Dutt, who holds exactly this type of conversation with executives through her work as founder and director of the global initiative Inter-Connected, finds that the discourse leads many to reexamine their own well-being and become champions for a more balanced existence. "If individuals feel that and start to be able to shift, and they [are in] positions of influence, then the system can start to change," says Dutt.

Measurement can be used to establish accountability. Citing a truism allegedly coined by 20th-century engineer W. Edwards Deming, Gora Mboup, president and CEO of Global Observatory linking Research to Action (GORA) Corp, in the United States and Senegal, observed to Bellagio colleagues that "what gets measured gets done." From Deming onward, countless careers and institutions have been built (and a few dismantled) by the link between measurement and accountability. Measurement is how we know whether, or to what degree, the outcome for which we are responsible was achieved. When coupled with clear expectations and consequences, measurement of well-being leads people in positions of influence to evaluate whether specific priorities and actions are contributing to or impeding well-being. These measurement roles are not unique to the realm of the well-being framework. There are, however, some dimensions of well-being measurement that require extra attention to make the metrics meaningful. These include what we measure, how we decide what to measure, how we conduct measurement, and how we interpret the data to distill meaning and inspire change.

Making Measures Meaningful

Well-being measures combine objective, subjective, and environmental indicators. The basic problem with measurement, as sociologist William Bruce Cameron wrote in 1963, is that not everything that can be counted counts, and not everything that counts can be counted.[17] Rita Giacaman, professor at Birzeit University's Institute of Community and Public Health in Palestine, paraphrased this statement in Bellagio when she urged colleagues to combine multiple measures and methodologies. Well-being measures address this challenge, determining ways to bring tangible data to intangible conditions and to elevate the "things that matter," by creating and tracking a broad set of indicators. Well-being measures combine objective indicators of conditions and subjective indicators of how people feel in the moment and about their lives overall. (Please refer to the **Figure** in the Introduction of this volume for an overview of well-being indicators.)

Subjective measures provide a more complete and contextualized under-standing of well-being than objective indicators alone; as the OECD's guidance observes, "A nation of materially wealthy, healthy, but miserable citizens is not the kind of place where most people would want to live."[18] Thus, for instance, subjective measures of perceived social connectedness or lack of connectedness might add context to objective measures such as voting rates. And, by drawing from multiple fields, subjective measures can produce a more nuanced under-standing of well-being. This adds "a multiplier effect" to the indicators' value "because of convergence into other areas, which greatly strengthens the im-pact on the individual," suggests Bellagio participant Anita Rajan, CEO of Tata STRIVE in India.

Yet, relying only on subjective measures of happiness would run the risk of creating the same "reductive view of the world" that comes from consid-ering only economic factors, notes Carrie Exton, head of OECD's Section for Monitoring Well-Being and Progress.

Bellagio participants observed that subjective measures also can be hard to interpret accurately, especially when people who live in objectively difficult situations, such as residents of Palestine, adapt to their circumstances—an ob-servation discussed more fully in this chapter's section on interpreting measure-ment data. The economist Sir Angus Deaton demonstrated another dimension of this problem in 2008 when he used subjective data from the Gallup World Poll to examine life satisfaction and health outcomes. Deaton found that the preva-lence of HIV appeared to have "little or no effect" on the proportion of people who were dissatisfied with their health,[19] and policymakers who relied on those findings alone may have thought there was no need to take action against HIV.[20]

Julia Kim, program director of the GNH Centre Bhutan, told those at the Bellagio convening that she sees an opportunity not to dethrone one type of measure in favor of another, but to help "ordinary people and politicians" understand what the indicators do and do not measure and what inequities they may mask. In Bhutan, for example, the GNH index is about balancing the outer and inner conditions for happiness; reconnecting to oneself, others, and nature; and creating the enabling conditions for happiness. As the first prime minister of Bhutan, Jigme Y. Thinley, put it, "true abiding happiness cannot exist while others suffer, but comes only from serving others, living in harmony with nature, and realizing our innate wisdom and the true and brilliant nature of our own mind," Kim explains.

We cannot talk about well-being in isolation from our relationship to the natural world.

—Julia Kim
Program Director
GNH Centre Bhutan

By including ecological diversity and resilience in its measures of happiness, Bhutan shifts us from an anthropocentric measurement framework, which focuses primarily on the human condition, to an ecocentric one, in which the natural world itself has *intrinsic* value, above and beyond its utility as a natural resource. This holistic approach to well-being is attracting attention from countries around the world, in the wake of climate changes and other environmental crises. But Indigenous cultures have cared about environmental measures for centuries; in fact, a common attribute of native populations across North America, Latin America, Australia, and New Zealand is that their conception of human well-being is interconnected with the well-being of the environment, according to Walter Flores, executive director of the Center for the Study of Equity and Governance in Health Systems, based in Guatemala and working globally.

The relational nature of well-being leads some thought leaders to wonder whether measuring the quality of "relationships"—among people; between employers and employees; between humans, their built environment, and nature; and between current and future generations—could lead to a deeper understanding of well-being. "Maybe if we [make] relationships a unit of analysis, then we can start really talking about health and address all the disconnection and alienation," suggests Katherine Trebeck, knowledge and policy lead for the global Wellbeing Economy Alliance.

Well-being measures illuminate root causes and early indicators of stressors and inequities as well as their downstream results. Building on the movement to address social determinants of health—the underlying social conditions from education to health care access to community conditions that affect people's ability to reach their best health—the well-being framework recognizes that health exists on a continuum from "ease" to "disease," as Rita Giacaman, professor at Birzeit University's Institute of Community and Public Health in Palestine, puts it. A person's path from one to the other is rarely direct; opportunities exist along the way to prevent disease (or unhappiness, or ill-being) before it becomes a full-blown condition. Attention to these "upstream" indicators also recognizes that barriers to health and well-being often are systemic, and therefore require systemic measurement and responses.

These indicators will vary greatly—and must be defined, measured, and addressed uniquely—depending on cultural, social, and political context. For example, in Palestine, some of the barriers to well-being exist at the intersection of the objective and subjective realm. These include factors that cause suffering, such as exposure to political violence, humiliation, human insecurity, violation of human rights, and racism. "We believe that it is ultimately the *political* determinants of health that determine the social determinants of health," Giacaman says. So, when thinking about well-being indicators, "we talk about all sorts of things like market forces, neoliberalism, biopower, biopolitics, necropolitics . . . country policies, global policies, and even factionalism within countries. All are political determinants which determine the social determinants and, along with biological predisposition, can lead to disease."

Much more work is needed to develop measures of equity. As chapter 1 underscored, equity is such a central factor that it could be considered a meta-indicator for all dimensions of well-being. Yet, even when metrics attempt to capture differences in equity or inclusion (e.g., by race, gender, or income) they tend to measure it in terms of representation rather than power, and the two are not the same. As Mao Amis, founder and executive director of the African Centre for a Green Economy, said in Bellagio, in post-apartheid South Africa black South Africans gained greater access to universities but the quality of their participation was constrained. And South African businesses began to give women more representation in the workplace, but they failed to transform the system in ways that would empower either women or blacks. Therefore, although representation changed, racial equity did not, Amis said. Better measures of equity would delve into the historic and structural impacts of exclusion, oppression, and marginalization on some groups and their impact on well-being. For example, residential segregation, rates of incarceration, and the mortality risks associated with pollution all reflect impacts of structural racism and inequity.

The challenge of measuring equity is complicated by the fact that measurement systems are built and controlled by the dominant, power-holding sectors of society. In that respect, says Mboup, the discussion about equity indicators is not only about measurement, but also about how we conceptualize well-being.

> We have to agree first that when you are living in a place of inequity, well-being will be affected. Measurement is the end goal, but the process is qualitative.
>
> —Gora Mboup
> President and CEO
> Global Observatory linking Research to Action (GORA) Corp
> United States and Senegal

Who is involved in defining and selecting measures matters. Éloi Laurent, senior economist at the Sciences Po Centre for Economic Research in France, asked his colleagues in Bellagio to recall the criticism leveled at a world-class commission that French President Nicholas Sarkozy formed in 2008 to examine how the wealth and social progress of a nation could be measured without relying on GDP. Economist Joseph Stiglitz chaired the Commission on the Measurement of Economic Performance and Social Progress, Amartya Sen served as its economic adviser, and Jean-Paul Fitoussi was the coordinator. The roster of the 25-member commission reads like a Who's Who of award winners in the economic world; in addition to the three leaders, it also included Kenneth Arrow, Anthony Atkinson, Angus Deaton, James J. Heckman, Daniel Kahneman, Robert Putnam, and others. The commission's findings, released a year later, made a big splash worldwide, as Stiglitz warned that "what we measure affects what we do. If we have the wrong metrics, we will strive for the wrong things. In the quest to increase GDP, we may end up with a society in which most citizens have become worse off."[21]

Yet, Laurent said, the commission's work was faulted "for not involving people in communities enough, and for just being a place where experts—in this case, Nobel Prize winners—gathered and decided, in a sense, for the people, what they should care about and what would be the best indicator" of well-being.

The criticism of the Stiglitz-Sen-Fitoussi commission echoed a broader dissatisfaction with who gets to decide what counts. "There are political and economic assumptions behind measures. There are cultural constructs behind measures. The numbers reflect a lot of historical complexity, and in some cases bias about the way one thinks the world works," observes Alonzo Plough, chief science officer and vice president of the Robert Wood Johnson Foundation.

In order to make measures meaningful, they should be developed in a way where they are meaningful to the populations we want to be better off than they are now.

—Alonzo Plough
Chief Science Officer and Vice President
Research-Evaluation-Learning
Robert Wood Johnson Foundation
United States

Involve the people whose conditions and experiences are being assessed in selecting and customizing measures. Traditional measurement models, created by traditional power holders, tend to be "riddled with white privilege," as Zeidler and others point out. Given the importance of cultural context, experiences, power dynamics, and other factors that affect well-being, it is crucial to involve the people and communities who are the subject of measurement in selecting, creating, and customizing measures so they align with their cultural traditions, values, priorities, and contexts. (Children and young people, who have their own voice and views about well-being, are among the populations to consult about what to measure; efforts in Nova Scotia and other places are exploring how to engage youth in their approaches.)

"Whenever [my team] comes up with a good idea, I ask, 'Will this make as much sense to the most marginalized citizen as it does to the mayor?' If it does, it's in. If it doesn't, it's not," Zeidler says.

Beginning in 2011, Trebeck led an effort by Oxfam Scotland to develop the Oxfam Humankind Index that measures multidimensional well-being. In collaboration with Strathclyde University, the New Economics Foundation, and others, Trebeck's team spent a year engaging with almost 3,000 people across Scotland to learn what they needed to live well in their communities.[22] Through polls, focus groups, street stalls, community workshops, and an online survey, the team made a special effort to reach "seldom heard" and marginalized communities, including African refugees and low-income workers. They ultimately identified 18 domains of factors that contribute to well-being, ranging from health and housing security to good relationships with family and friends, access to green and social spaces, access to arts and culture, having good transportation, being part of a community, and so on.[22] The developers then weighted the domains according to the importance that emerged via the consultation and matched them to the best available measures from publicly accessible databases.

"Much to our surprise, [the Humankind Index] punched way above its weight in terms of challenging the politics around what Scottish success was, what the role of government was, and what the purpose of the economy should be—an independent evaluation bears this out," Trebeck told colleagues in Bellagio. Her takeaway: Taking time to include communities and put people's voices at the forefront makes sense not only because it is more ethical and produces more relevant content, but because it is strategically useful.

> It's very hard for politicians to not take notice of something when you say, "This is what a huge number of the population really wants."
>
> —Katherine Trebeck
> Knowledge and Policy Lead
> Wellbeing Economy Alliance
> Scotland

Indigenous peoples are especially important co-creators when measures are being developed. There are about 370 million Indigenous people in the world, belonging to 5,000 different groups and spread across 90 countries worldwide.[23] That's a population too big to ignore if we want to advance a global well-being framework, Flores reminded Bellagio participants. And yet, these people often *are* ignored, by policymakers and by developers of measurement systems. This is problematic for equity reasons, and also because in many more ecocentric cultures, priorities often lie in protecting the environment and sovereign territories and ensuring intergenerational equity rather than accumulating wealth.

Using Measurement Tools Effectively

There is an old Romanian saying, "A bad workman blames his tools." The French put their own twist on it: "A bad workman never *finds* a good tool." Both are probably right. But it was the American academician Father John Culkin who really nailed the connection between humans and the constructs they use to make sense of the world: "We shape our tools, and then our tools shape us."

Measures are tools, and even with all the right processes to select all the right measures, if those tools aren't used well they can result in a distorted or incomplete understanding of well-being. To date, most well-being research has focused on refining measurement, in the belief that it is possible to change what is measured. How can measures continue to become more relevant, while also being directly applied to shift narratives and mindsets, and to create meaningful action by communities and policymakers? Bellagio participants had several ideas.

Use fewer and sharper measures, but avoid reducing them to a single number that signifies "well-being." Governments and media often push to have one number they can use to assess the current state of well-being, progress toward greater well-being, and how well-being in one place compares with that of another. It is true that keeping measurement simple helps to tell a clearer story, and it's true that the array of metrics could use some pruning to produce a set that is comparable, contextual, diverse, robust, authoritative, and ideally not in silos, Bellagio participants decided during a small-group discussion. Still, any measurement of well-being encompasses a huge number of complex, interrelated variables, and boiling them down causes much of the story to evaporate. "Even though it's tempting to come up with a nice, jazzy number . . . really try to avoid simplifying it too much," Zeidler advised.

Avoid reinforcing old paradigms of value when trying to quantify well-being. In the effort to make a compelling case for why well-being matters and why it is worth investing in, people often try to monetize the value. Tools have been developed to try to capture and describe well-being's worth, or some proxy for it. Economists and government planners, for instance, often use the value of a statistical life, which is defined as the additional cost that individuals would be willing to bear for changes that, in the aggregate, reduce the expected number of fatalities by one.[24] Measuring well-being this way is problematic, however, because it tends to give more value to the life of someone who is rich than to someone who is poor. When organizations like OECD compare the value of a statistical life across countries, Laurent observes, the life of an American appears to be four times more "valuable" than the life of someone in China because the flow of wages and economic wealth created by an American is presumed to be much higher than those created by a Chinese person.

How can measurement approaches frame health and well-being as assets that individuals and companies appreciate and want to invest in? Or, as Amis asked colleagues in Bellagio, "If money is the currency of the world, how can we use money to achieve our agenda of building a well-being economy?" There have been efforts to attach monetary values to components of well-being. Well Worth, developed by Happy City, translated well-being into quantifiable impacts on education, health, and other domains. (Well Worth is not used today because it requires continual updating, a major undertaking.) Another approach is to measure the loss of quality of life due to ill-being or ill health, and then calculate the treatment costs as a percentage of overall social spending.

A third approach assigns different weights (calculated in monetary terms) to various determinants of well-being. Thus, a divorce (or a particular health status, etc.) would be worth X dollars of life satisfaction/well-being. This approach, called income equivalence, is a way to gauge relative magnitudes and differences in well-being, according to Carol Graham, Leo Pasvolsky senior fellow at the Brookings Institution and a professor at the University of Maryland. Participants at Bellagio cautioned that by defining and valuing well-being in economic terms, the discussion and measurement of well-being support and further reinforce an economics-only concept of progress.

Conversely, there have been efforts to attach well-being values to monetary terms. In 2017, the Happy City initiative mounted a campaign, #InvestInHappy, that aimed to expand popular notions of "investment" beyond monetary connotations to also include time, love, attention, and skills, and to get people to place more value on interactions with friends, family, communities, and natural resources. The campaign's goal was to facilitate 30,000 online conversations and 600 workshops and workplace trainings.[25]

Capture the stories behind the data. Just as measurement requires *both* objective and subjective measures, and just as a single number cannot provide sufficient nuance to explain well-being, the stories behind the numbers are essential for understanding what the numbers mean. And well-being metrics yield infinitely more stories than purely economic measures by unpacking the experiences, perceptions, conditions, and realities that eventually manifest as outcome data. The stories explain what the conditions are that advance or diminish well-being, and how those conditions and experiences affect well-being. In Bellagio, a small-group discussion about measurement generated consensus that "It [is] a real [risk] often that we just talk about the data," Zeidler reported to the full gathering. "We need the stories of change. We need the stories of need. We need the stories of individual differences. When you use well-being as a framework, what are the stories that those metrics are telling us?"

Fietje called this interplay between numeric values and narrative complexity a "wonderful, powerful conversation" that tells us what happens at the individual, family, and community level. Dutt further explains: "Whether it's life or death, or nutrition, or access to health or education, or the consequences of violence upon your person . . . storytelling [shifts what] we could be addressing" through policy change.

Interpreting Data to Make Meaning and Inspire Change

Kim reminded Bellagio colleagues that Simon Kuznets, the economist-statistician who created the tools for measuring gross national product in 1934, famously had qualms about how the numbers might be interpreted. "No income measurement undertakes to estimate the reverse side of income, that is, the intensity and unpleasantness of effort going into the earning of income," he wrote in the Commerce Department's report to Congress. "The welfare of a nation can, therefore, scarcely be inferred from a measurement of national income."[26] This chapter has established that economic indicators and non-economic indicators should be combined to accurately measure well-being. But even so, how can data be safely interpreted to make the measures meaningful? Bellagio participants offer this advice.

Consider the desired narrative. In ways discussed more fully in section 3, how measurements are interpreted reflects, and also drives, the broader narrative about what matters, how to define progress, and why to measure well-being in the first place. What is the desired paradigm shift? Is the goal just to take the temperature, as Fietje says—to understand what the state of well-being is at this point of time? Or is it to be able to say something about growth—and, if so, growth for what purpose? If not economic growth, then what kind?

Is it that everyone should be happier? If so, how much is enough, and is more always better? Analyses of data spanning the fields of biology, genetics, psychology, and economics show that, on average, people who have higher levels of well-being do better over time. "They invest more because they believe in their futures," Carol Graham explains. "Because of that, they do better; they lead longer, healthier, happier lives. [So] it isn't necessarily that we want more and more and more" well-being. It's because well-being "really does matter to people's lives, individually [and] in the collective."

Often, Fietje says, the "shades of gray" that arise from interpreting well-being data are more interesting than coming up with any singular number. Data analysts in Bhutan might agree. In that country, which has a largely Buddhist culture, the narrative about well-being encompasses the idea of contentment and finding balance between material and spiritual needs, Kim explains. Policymakers analyze data from the annual Gross National Happiness survey not to figure out how to make those who are already happy happier, but to understand who is falling below the sufficiency threshold and, subsequently, what changes are needed to increase their well-being. "How we define sufficiency . . . what is the narrative of success, these things are all part of the story" of which data interpretation is one part, Kim says.

Disaggregate data to gain a true picture of well-being at the subpopulation level. Measurement experts urge going "below the skin of what the numbers can tell us" to deepen the analysis of well-being. By digging down into the variation among different groups in society and looking for their possible causes—including political and economic assumptions, cultural constructs, and historical complexities—the analysis and interpretation of data can uncover inequities. "Your metric, on its own, might not tell you that there is a historical [basis for inequity] going on here, but your analysis definitely should be picking that through," says Exton. In the most recent GNH survey in Bhutan, for instance, analysts found that women overall reported lower happiness levels than men, and farmers lower levels than other occupations, identifying those groups as a priority for further analysis and, potentially, interventions.

Ensure that subjective measures of well-being neither mask nor excuse inequities, if people in objectively poor conditions report high levels of well-being. As Carol Graham pointed out in the previous chapter, people are extremely adaptable. A very poor person in ill health may profess satisfaction with his or her health, not because they are happy with being ill, but because they have adapted to living that way and have no expectation of becoming well. Bellagio participant Mboup related this to his own lived experience: "When you have hope, you build resilience," he said. "And that is very important. In my case, before me, my mother lost four children. Later, because I did my PhD on infant mortality, I knew it was because of poverty. But despite all those things, they taught us to be resilient. That is [why] I always tell people I have never felt I was poor. It's just when I grew up and I analyzed data, I understood that my situation was a situation of poverty."

This makes data interpretation complicated; it is important not to undervalue the assets in communities that make their subjective well-being level high, but consideration also must be given to whether the level reported by respondents merely reflects adaptation to a state of ill-being or inequity. Carol Graham suggests using vignettes and other survey methods to test differences in how people of different cultures, races, gender, and income levels answer well-being questions, and adjusting the interpretation accordingly.

Offer different layers of information to help make meaning. "Individual indicators measure one specific thing," Zeidler says, "but when you bring them together into a domain or subdomain, they tell a story and help support change." Zeidler describes three layers of information used to report the data from the Thriving Places Index:

- *Headline-level information* shapes public discourse: "Are we creating the local conditions for people to thrive, and doing so equitably and fairly?"
- *Mid-level information* includes the sub-domains that make sense of that headline—What do we mean by "local conditions"?—and let people see their part in it. This may mean more detailed information on education and learning, work and economy, community and environment, and other factors. For example, "Is the local economy supporting local people and businesses?"
- *Detailed information* gets into the indicators themselves, giving the granular detail needed to actually use the metrics to measure change, to prioritize action, to learn what works, to see strengths and needs, and to assess impact. For example: "Are the jobs being created in the local economy providing people with work that is reasonably secure, paying a living wage, and leaving them neither under- or overworked?"

Examine the gaps between measures. Even when a nation's economy is booming, well-being data might show widespread, premature deaths. Or, as happened in China, life satisfaction might plummet despite a decade of rapid economic growth. The gaps between standard economics-based measures and more comprehensive measures of well-being, in particular, are good at raising "interesting questions that point us in the direction of better understanding the deeper dimensions of well-being," Carol Graham suggests.

Examine biases in metrics and analysis. Depending on who is designing and analyzing well-being measures, and the assumptions, power, and worldview they bring to the process, results can vary greatly. For instance, the assumption that some countries are more developed than others, and that all should want to become more developed, influences the meaning analysts will take from measures of economic, social, and environmental change. It is important to question those assumptions, especially to determine whether an analysis is based on a Western-centric interpretation of value that ignores conceptions of well-being from an Indigenous, first-peoples' viewpoint. Romlie Mokak, CEO of the Lowitja Institute, a Djugun man and member of the Yawuru people in Australia, calls for a focused effort to "decolonize data . . . [meaning] to really be clear about the biases that exist not only in the . . . metrics but really at the substantive level of the analysis."

Ensure that marginalized groups are not viewed solely in terms of deficits. Mokak's institute is deeply involved in trying to change the deficit-based conversation about Aboriginal and Torres Strait Islander peoples. "It's about the gap. It's about disparity. It's about dysfunction. It's about disadvantage," Mokak says.

> *This deficit discourse becomes correlated with problematic people. This becomes internalized with our people, and that's the future that young people often see: What gets reflected back in the mirror is deficit and despair.*
> *—Romlie Mokak*
> *CEO*
> *Lowitja Institute*
> *Australia*

Although it is important to note gaps in well-being from an equity perspective, it is just as important to interpret well-being measures with an emphasis on cultural strengths.

Ensure a participatory approach, giving local people control over their data and how it is interpreted and used. Echoing the earlier discussion about involving communities in defining measures, it is also imperative to work with— and share power with—people at the grassroots level to interpret the meaning and the policy implications of data. Importantly, those data belong to the community, and the community must have a say in how they are used or shared. This is often referred to as data sovereignty, particularly regarding the individual and collective right of Indigenous peoples to control data from and about their communities and lands.

Next Steps for Measurement

There is no doubt that measurement is a powerful tool—for providing insights into well-being, for informing policies, for changing the narrative. What we measure, who determines what to measure, how we measure, and how we interpret data all have a profound impact on social change. In this regard, well-being is more than a measurement of human conditions; it is a way of thinking, understanding, and taking action.

The good news is that social scientists, economists, and others have made considerable progress in identifying new measures, fixing flawed measures, and identifying others to develop further. People now know more than ever before about how to assess and evaluate well-being. But there also is no doubt that the practice of measuring well-being still needs improvement. Although some determinants of well-being are consistent across countries, cultures, individuals, and time, many others vary greatly and require new techniques to capture them. More must be done to demonstrate the value of these new measures and to devise practical solutions based on the data they provide. It still isn't clear exactly how to measure civil society or adaptive systems, for example. People are just beginning to learn how well-being affects the interactions among biological, psychological, and genetic components. And there is much more to do to address the power dynamics that affect measurement and the misalignment between what people say matters to them and what happens as a result of political and economic systems.

What lies ahead? More work to fine-tune measures and to link the field of well-being with the measurement of related concepts, such as resilience. More involvement of diverse community groups in discussions about well-being measures and initiatives. More effort to translate people's views, values, and wishes into the decision-making structures, at every level of authority.

Most of all, it's important not to wait for the perfect measures before taking action to create change. "There can be a real wish to get the questionnaire perfect, or to get all the indicators right, but actually . . . there will be room to fix it as you go along," Kim reminds us. "So don't let perfection be the enemy of the good."

SECTION III

NARRATIVES AND CULTURE

People understand information, shape their priorities, and justify or change their decisions in part through their narratives, the shared ideas that help them make meaning of their world. Built on the underlying and often unspoken beliefs that comprise cultures, narratives influence people's interpretation of how things are, how things should be, and what is better or worse. They are built over time, and are often sustained by a dominant group in order to institutionalize and maintain its power. Shifting narratives, then—in alignment with culture, cultural context, and cultural identity—is a powerful tool for social change and transformations in power structures.

Narrative was an overarching topic of conversation at the Bellagio gathering. The group repeatedly circled back to the need and opportunity to change the narrative that defines progress and for an authentic well-being narrative to gain currency. Narrative change was the focus of two case studies, from Nova Scotia and Singapore, and played a leading role in all of the on-the-ground work shared by the group.

The challenge is that during this last century, the dominant narratives in much of the world have largely equated progress and power with wealth and consumption, fueled by reliance on economic measures, as discussed in section 2. While the postwar era that has focused on GDP and other economic indicators has driven significant progress—global reductions of poverty; increased access to water, food, and education; increased life expectancy; and many others—it has also established a narrative of progress that is too narrow. This narrative has failed to help us see, understand, or adequately address increases in inequity, grave disparities in lived experiences, unsustainable draws on natural capital, and serious damage to intergenerational prosperity.

Changing this narrative to one centered on well-being and equity holds great promise, and efforts to do so must align closely with cultural context. Culture, including the ability to connect with and fully express one's cultural identity, is a significant component of well-being. And efforts to define and pursue well-being must be done in alignment with cultural context. For example, in New Zealand, well-being measures were based on the OECD's Better Life Index, modified with input from the community, including Māori leaders, to integrate specific cultural priorities, such as the intrinsic connection between well-being of land and people. Without this, the measures would not be able to gain currency or accurately measure well-being.

Any new narrative will need to emerge from deep grassroots engagement and connect with values relevant to each community. It will need to overcome the dominance of existing narratives that are widely known and reinforced on a constant basis by media, pop culture and entertainment, the marketplace, policy framing, political speech, and many other factors. And while changing narratives can help to advance changes in expectations, shifts in power dynamics, and experimentation, it also can spark opposition from entrenched institutions and those who benefit from the status quo. The work of developing, stewarding, and advancing a well-being narrative, while complex, is critical to advancing well-being.

Chapter 5, "Capturing the Cultural Narratives of Well-Being," by Bellagio participant Nils Fietje and his colleague Felicity Thomas from the World Health Organization (WHO), explores the importance of cultural context in defining and making sense of narratives; the way narratives often reflect and perpetuate existing power structures; and the potential for narratives to shift perspectives, power dynamics, and cultural expectations.

Chapter 6, "The Power of Shifting Narratives, Expectations, and Consciousness: Discussion and Case Studies From Bellagio," follows the thread of narrative through every aspect of the discourse at Bellagio, including why narrative matters; how a shift in narrative can be a lever to advance change; the importance of grassroots engagement and framing with authentic cultural context; and other key considerations that will impact how a new narrative is developed, tested, refined, and applied.

Shifting the narrative about what progress means and building currency and relevance for a well-being framing is a fundamental pathway to drive changes in policy and practice—and to ultimately reshape the shared expectations of society.

Capturing the Cultural Narratives of Well-Being

FELICITY THOMAS, PHD*

Senior Research Fellow, University of Exeter, United Kingdom

NILS FIETJE, PHD*

Research Officer, Regional Office for Europe, World Health Organization, Denmark

Measures of national income and gross domestic product (GDP) have long been at the center of narratives[†] of country-level "success." While this economic narrative continues to enjoy extensive influence around the globe, a look at the origins of GDP itself reminds us that it developed out of a particular historical and cultural context. Arising from the United States of America depression of the 1930s and the economic pressures of World War II, GDP was originally developed to measure economic production and to prepare Western nations better for warfare. Despite this, and its clear American-Anglo origins, the political economy of the day meant its influence spread widely—first as a template for accounting that all nations wishing to receive postwar aid under America's Marshall Plan were required to abide by, and second through its adoption by the United States-based World Bank and International Monetary Fund as a standard tool for measuring— and assessing the worth of—national economies.[1] As a result, a Western-led definition of progress and success, which placed focus on the economics of production—rather than on issues such as welfare, environmental pollution, health inequalities, and care—soon became a prescribed means of measurement

---

† Those subjective stories that help us make sense of our subjective experiences.

for countries around the globe, and has been translated in popular meaning and narrative, from the worth of economies to the worth of nations and communities.

In recent decades, however, widespread recognition of flaws and limitations in GDP measures have resulted in the development of a range of alternative approaches to evaluate societal success. The Report of the Commission on the Measurement of Economic Performance and Social Progress (aka the Stiglitz Report 2009) in particular has played a pivotal role in recommending ways of moving beyond dominant GDP measures to capture data on subjective well-being.[2] With its overall concern on "what counts for common people's well-being" and with the most important features that give life its value, its boldest departure from conventional approaches is its aim to measure people's *own* assessment of their well-being and quality of life. Influenced by the head of the commission, Amartya Sen, the report draws on a capability and freedoms approach,[3]* as well as Aristotelian concepts of eudaimonia,† in which "true happiness is found in the expression of virtue—that is, in doing what is worth doing."[4]

The comparison of well-being with GDP that has resulted following this and other reports has been both a blessing and a curse. On the one hand, it has created an important space where the dominant Western-led narrative of progress as a function of economic success can be challenged. At the same time, however, it has arguably led to a false expectation that, like GDP, well-being must be expressed numerically. One only has to look to the burgeoning of indices intent on identifying measurements of "happiness" or "quality of life" (e.g., OECD Better Life Index, the World Happiness Report, the World Values Survey, the Gallup World Poll, the Happy Planet Index) to see that dominant paradigms remain fixed on quantitative measurements that emphasize individualized and often hedonistic notions of well-being‡ that create and fuel a particular narrative around individual responsibility and societal achievement. Reducing an entire country's economic output to a robust, comparable, and meaningful set of digits is challenging enough. But at least the variables are inherently numeric. For well-being, a rich tapestry of social behaviors, cultural contexts, and historical beliefs have to be reduced to a set of quantitative measurements that can quickly become so abstracted as to lose all meaning, if not beauty.

Furthermore, while research on subjective well-being can provide an array of metrics around happiness or life satisfaction, their focus on individual psychology means that what the data really show, and the way that they are understood within the broader context of a person's life, is very often overlooked. In

---

* The core focus of the capability approach is on what individuals are able to do.

† Eudaimonic well-being has a rich history of definitions. As a philosophical concept, it is often traced back to Aristotle. More recently, it has been employed in the positive psychology movement. In general, definitions often include aspects of autonomy, competence, purpose of life, and control.

‡ Hedonic well-being is based on the notion that increased pleasure and decreased pain lead to happiness.

their qualitative research on well-being in Bangladesh, for example, Devine and White (2013) found that it was difficult to separate out ideas on well-being from moral and religious discourse about the way things were and should be. This, they argued, suggests that "having a good life" may be seen as less important than "*living* a good life," and reminds us that existing narratives around well-being are heavily reflective of the academic disciplines, and indeed the basic human cultural contexts, that underpin them.[5]

Narratives of well-being are influenced by the tools that we use to make sense of well-being. Very often, such tools are designed by academics imposing discipline-focused conceptualizations around what counts as "data" and "evidence," despite the difficulties many people are known to experience abstracting the complexity of their lives into simple scores relating to notions such as "happiness" and "satisfaction." Notwithstanding its ongoing and widespread use, for example, the conceptualizations underpinning the survey tool Cantril's Ladder—with its culturally loaded implication of striving and of climbing a ladder, as well as its idea of "complete satisfaction" with life—has been found to be problematic.[6] Quantitative measurements also tend to overlook socio-cultural norms, expectations, and aspirations around well-being and life satisfaction. In some areas, reported high levels of satisfaction may, for example, mask political oppression or simply the wish to "save face" or look good, rather than any genuinely positive experience.[7] Understandings around what constitutes a good life can also be swayed by changing societal norms and expectations, complicating attempts to compare well-being across time and space.

Dominant narratives of well-being not only influence how it is conceptualized, but may in turn have implications for the kinds of research and intervention that take place, particularly when theories of behavior and "success" are utilized that see Western ideals as the "gold standard." It is also worth noting that much of the energy driving the current well-being agenda has derived from the Global North, and from those who are already in a position of relative advantage. Seen in this way, it is necessary to ask how the ideas embedded within the concept of well-being itself (stressing individualized and capitalist ideologies of choice, consumption, aspiration, and morality) may themselves reflect a Western construct, and how this narrative may or may not have value in other parts of the world.

However sophisticated and seductive existing measurements of well-being might be, it is clear that they alone cannot, and will not, achieve the changes to policy and practice that are necessary to improve and sustain well-being for all. To do so requires a paradigm shift away from individualized and often Western-centric notions that emphasize an economic narrative, to more contextualized, culturally informed, and relational understandings and narratives of well-being.

In this chapter, we attempt to show how a greater awareness of people's lived experience can shape a more robust well-being narrative that offers policymakers greater insight into what matters to the good life of their rich and varied publics.

Changing the Cultural Narrative on Well-Being

Recent years have seen a number of initiatives and publications emerge to support a new kind of narrative on well-being. Among the most influential is a call for "fifth wave" thinking.[8,9] This recognizes that existing, individually focused, and biomedical approaches to health and well-being are no longer amenable to the challenges of the current era, and that a radically new approach—the fifth wave—that focuses on "a culture for health" and that seeks to engage with the full complexity of subjective, lived experience is needed to address contemporary problems, such as social inequality and loss of well-being. See **Figure 1**.

Figure 1. The fifth wave of public health improvement—a culture for health[10]

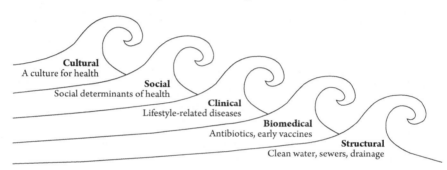

Although grounded in public health and originally based on the historical context of the United Kingdom, fifth-wave thinking may provide a useful way of conceptualizing well-being, which enables a shift away from individualized responsibility toward a more contextualized, collective, and relational approach. Recognizing the need to "adopt a new image of what it means to be human,"[11] this approach recognizes individual and societal assets, and fosters a greater sense of empathy and compassion within society so that the "diseases" of modern society (depression, obesity, inequality, etc.) are framed not as individual failings, but as *collective* issues that require collective responses.

Drawing on such thinking to create a new well-being-based cultural narrative is, of course, no mean feat, and will almost certainly be imbued with political and economic ramifications and relations of power. Yet, despite the challenges, narratives can and do change. A change in thinking and narrative relating to tobacco use (from "individual decision and right to smoke" to "deceitful tobacco industry practices, and collective harms from second-hand smoke and tobacco-related illness") has evolved across much of the globe in recent decades, with a range of positive implications for health and well-being. As the example in Box 1 illustrates, tapping into universal values, such as the sanctity of the child, can

---

Box 1 **Shifting the Cultural Narrative on Smoking in Thailand**

"Can I get a light?" was the question children asked that shocked adult smokers in Thailand, eliciting a stream of reasons from the adults why the children should not light up. Unknown to the adults, the children were actors for an award-winning campaign video created by Ogilvy and Mather for the Thai Health Promotion Foundation.*

Prior to this, strict tobacco legislation and regulation, heavy investment in scare-tactic anti-smoking commercials, and a Quitline to help people stop smoking had yielded few results. With a budget of just $5,000, the Smoking Kid campaign generated widespread attention, and a substantial and sustained increase in calls to the Quitline, outperforming all other anti-smoking campaigns in the country in the past 20 years. The key to its success was the way it changed the narrative on smoking by convincing people to reflect on their actions at a personal level, and to set a positive example to the younger generation. The video sparked widespread conversations among smokers and non-smokers within Thailand and beyond and made the support available to quit more visible.[11]

---

help surface unconscious biases and nudge a deeply ingrained narrative about personal freedom toward one of collective responsibility.

This example also demonstrates how different types of narrative have the potential for very different well-being outcomes that require different policy and practice interventions to improve well-being. Recognition of this lies at the heart of the work of the World Health Organization (WHO) Regional Office for Europe, whose Cultural Contexts of Health and Well-Being (CCH) project aims to highlight how our experiences and narratives of well-being and health are fundamentally influenced by the cultural contexts from which we make meaning.[†] These frameworks, WHO recognizes, inform the beliefs and actions of policymakers, health care practitioners, and other actors in the private and nongovernmental organization (NGO) sectors as much as the people they serve. For this reason, the project promotes the idea that policymakers must seek not only to understand the values they attribute to others, but also to critically

---

* The award-winning video for the Thai Health Promotion Foundation can be found at *www. youtube.com/watch? v=g_YZ_ptMKw0*

† For more information about the CCH project, see *www.euro.who.int/en/cch*

Box 2 **Winning Hearts and Minds on Marriage Equality**

In the United States, the Civil Marriage Collaborative (CMC) set the stage for the 2015 ruling by the Supreme Court to make marriage equality the law of the land by fundamentally shifting the narrative on the subject. Important work to advance marriage equality was happening at the grassroots level and by engaging elected officials, celebrities, and diverse organizations and champions. But research showed that the "equal rights and benefits" narrative being employed by advocates for marriage equality was reinforcing the belief that while heterosexual couples married for love, gay couples were driven by a different values frame: equality. Transitioning to a narrative grounded in reconnecting the narrative to the core, shared value of love (i.e., "love is love"), employing a different set of messengers (parents and grandparents of gay people), and working collaboratively to deliver the new narrative across the movement is one of the key components credited with making it possible to change hearts and minds on the subject of marriage equality, leading to the Supreme Court decision.[12]

---

examine their own cultures—their perceptions, daily practices, processes of decision-making, and the narratives that these uphold—and their effects on people who may or may not share the same values and priorities, and whose lived experiences and cultural context create different lenses through which narrative is received, processed, and applied.

The importance of grounding narratives in values—especially values that are shared across cultures—has been demonstrated time and again, as reflected in Box 2.

Other examples can be seen in the work of organizations whose very raison d'être is to challenge dominant narratives. The American Friends Service Committee,* for example, employs narrative change strategies to overturn dominant discourses that overdetermine how people understand important issues, such as Islamophobia, and the politics and everyday lives of people in Gaza. New Tactics in Human Rights[+] similarly seeks to foster alternative narratives that give voice to marginalized perspectives and create more possibility for social change, as shown in Box 3.

---

* For more information about the American Friends Service Committee, see *www.afsc.org*
+ For more information about New Tactics in Human Rights, see *www.newtactics.org*

Box 3 **Rewriting the Gender Narrative in Egypt**

Traditional folk stories are an important element of popular culture in Egypt, but they often communicate normative social beliefs about gender roles that marginalize women. The Women and Memory Forum (WMF) in Egypt started the Women's Stories project to enable women to rewrite traditional stories from their own perspectives. This allowed women to challenge traditional texts, increase awareness of gender rights, redefine their role in society, and develop their writing skills. The WMF has published some of the new versions of the stories produced by the women, and has translated them into public performances, enabling the materials to be disseminated to a wide audience. Following its success, the WMF has begun gender-sensitive story writing workshops for young Palestinian girls and in Sudan.[13]

Reshaping what counts as evidence

Key to moving forward is a shift in thinking away from singularly defined framings of well-being, to explore how accounts of these notions are produced and driven, and, perhaps, to allow for a more pluralistic understanding of the concept of well-being. Incorporating what are often marginalized or peripheral voices into discussion and decision-making is vital and requires serious attention to be given to forms of evidence that elicit the beliefs, practices, values, and social processes that can shape how well-being is understood and practiced. This means looking beyond quantitative measurements of well-being, and elevating the status of qualitative approaches in the traditional hierarchy of evidence, in order to make evidence generated from research methods, such as ethnography, focus groups, oral histories, or narrative approaches, more admissible to policy discourse.

Instead of rating other people against Western measurements of well-being, this means listening to how people think, feel, and describe their lives in their own words or images, and how they see this being affected by the terms on which other people and systems engage with them. Box 4 demonstrates clearly why localized perspectives on well-being must be prioritized over existing dominant paradigms of understanding.

Narrative research methods can provide insight into people's understandings of well-being, and their health and well-being-related experiences and lifestyle choices can locate this within their broader socio-cultural and historical context. At WHO, these approaches are central to the CCH project, and have informed

---

Box 4 **Socio-Cultural Barriers to Latrine Use in Odisha, India**

Open defecation is widely practiced in India. To improve sanitation and promote health and well-being, the Government of India has instituted large-scale sanitation programs supporting construction of public toilets and subsidizing household latrine buildings in rural areas. However, many latrines remain unused. Qualitative research was undertaken in Odisha, where latrine use was especially low. It found that practical issues (e.g., poor construction) and the need to carry water to the latrine acted as deterrents to use. Importantly, a range of culturally engrained norms also deterred people from latrine use. For women, open defecation alongside others was not only valued as a safe experience, but it provided an important daily opportunity for discussion, social bonding, and relaxing that was unavailable in the cramped latrines. The research emphasized the value of eliciting local perspectives and norms before implementing future sanitation programs.[14]

---

key documents, such as an award-winning Health Evidence Network report* authored by Professor Trish Greenhalgh, and a Profile on Health and Well-Being for Italy, which will form a template for narrative reporting on well-being across the WHO European Region. The latter report explores the degree to which the limits of quantitative well-being measurement can be supplemented by narrative research methods. This approach utilized a diverse set of sources, from popular literature to artistic outputs and social media, to uncover and explore how dominant well-being motifs (such as the fragmentation of the family, or the perception of the refugee crisis) are being played out in the context of Italy.

That these approaches are being taken seriously is at least in part due to their recognition in the *European Health Report 2015: Targets and Beyond—Reaching New Frontiers in Evidence*, which specifically states a need for countries to look beyond "facts and figures" to embrace evidence from the humanities and social sciences in order to meaningfully report on "what it means to be healthy and well in Europe."[15]

While these approaches provide a mechanism that facilitates diverse and inclusive understandings of well-being, collating and analyzing evidence of subjective experience and assimilating this meaningfully into well-being-related policy and practice is not without issue. It is important to recognize, for example,

---

* The report can be found at *http://www.euro.who.int/en/data-and-evidence/evidence-informed-policy-making/publications/2016/cultural-contexts-of-health-the-use-of-narrative-research-in-the-health-sector-2016*

that the kinds of narrative these methods and approaches produce will be heavily influenced by the voices that are heard—as well as those that are not. Furthermore, while the stories told through narratives can challenge norms, they can also reproduce dominant thinking, and can influence the way that people act, think, and relate to others, as well as what they aspire to and expect. One only has to recognize the power held by spin doctors in contemporary politics to realize that there is much to gain by holding charge over the narrative that is told. The intense focus within political rhetoric and popular media around blaming and shaming those living in poverty—a narrative that reinforces individual-level vs. societal-level action, or erodes support for any action at all—is an especially clear example of this across many neoliberally oriented contexts (see for example, Chase and Walker 2015).[16]

As has been well recognized within international development studies, "participatory" research and interventions aimed at improving well-being can also (albeit often inadvertently) officialize what are sometimes quite limited and skewed ranges of narratives without acknowledging the diversity of perspectives that exist within an assumed "community"—as described in an example in Box 5—again emphasizing the need to ensure that narratives around well-being are truly reflective of all.

Although qualitative methods can usefully help ensure that a diversity of voices can feed into the development of a well-being-based cultural narrative,

---

Box 5 **Authoritative Accounts of Well-Being**

Juan Loera-González's ethnographic work among the Ramamuri Indigenous people in Northern Mexico highlights the potential pitfalls involved when attempting to construct a narrative of "community" well-being. Introduced to the Ramamuri through the local leader, Loera-González was given access to informants in positions of power and influence. This led to the emergence of a dominant and homogenized narrative of well-being that was framed in terms of ethnic identity, and that emphasized and legitimated certain ways of thinking, while masking less visible variations and contradictions, and leaving out those more marginalized individuals who did not see eye-to-eye with the political leadership. Over time, and reflecting on the narrow version of well-being he was hearing, Loera-González was able to move away from his association with the dominant groups to listen to more hidden and non-legitimized perspectives of well-being held by young people, migrant workers, and individuals who did not support the political status quo.[17]

it is necessary to recognize that they do not, by themselves, necessarily contest the normative notions that underpin dominant paradigms. Used inappropriately, they too can serve to reproduce and fuel the very power relations that they seek to unsettle. For instance, grand narratives around local participation, accountability, democracy, and transparency are frequently used by those with power, precisely to carry out top-down, "expert"-driven interventions that benefit the status quo, rather than enabling any form of meaningful change.[18,19] As Greenhalgh (2016) points out, it is only through the "appropriate and rigorous use of narrative methods that diverse cultural contexts can be incorporated (or adequately responded to) in the policy-making process."[20]

Relational well-being

Realizing the potential of fifth-wave thinking requires a rich mix of perspectives and expertise that acknowledge the central role culture plays in the construction of well-being narratives. This in turn requires an approach that is shaped by all members of society—individuals, communities, academic institutions, local and national governments, civil society, the private sector, and the media. To help envisage how this may be achieved, Hinchliffe et al. (2018) draw upon the concept of "healthy publics." Rather than "public health"—seen to assume an already constituted public waiting passively to be informed and intervened upon—its inversion ("healthy publics") enables recognition of the need to work in a collective and engaged manner with those who have lived experience of, or the potential to have their lives influenced by, a particular well-being-related issue or intervention.[21]

At the heart of this thinking is recognition of the need to move away from individualized formulations, to approaches that recognize the value of *relational* well-being. While well-being is of course about personal processes and relationships, relational well-being recognizes that the personal is deeply intertwined with broader societal processes—including wealth disparities, economic forces, and the markers of social difference that are played out through constructions of gender, race, ethnicity, religion, age, sexuality, and dis/ability.

Seen in this way, it is clear that well-being is not something that we can "have" or obtain; rather it is something that happens or emerges in the interrelations between personal, societal, and environmental processes.[21] There is also increasing recognition that it is the interplay and interaction of different variables, in often unpredictable ways, that create stasis and degeneration, as well as important openings for new relationships which may provide vital "opportunity spaces" for transforming ways of thinking and working.[22,23]

It is also clear that to achieve a narrative inclusive of cultural variations in understanding, well-being requires a momentous shift in mindset away from dominant thinking in which "experts" are needed to "fix" what are perceived as problems—and a shift away from narratives that reinforce this status quo—to narratives that advance relational well-being and that mobilize and sustain a genuinely collective dialogue and effort toward well-being. For decades, costly interventions that seek to "fix" some of the most disadvantaged communities in which poverty, crime, unemployment, and poor health are rife have largely failed because they impose top-down, deficits-based thinking about those within them. This leads to a narrative that positions community members as "problems" and "risks" or as passive victims who need fixing or intervening upon in order to bring their behaviors and attitudes into line with what are regarded to be more accepted—and acceptable—ways of being.

Assets-based narratives

Alternative approaches that draw on the concept of salutogenesis* have gained traction over the past decade. Assets-based approaches are concerned with facilitating people and communities to come together to achieve positive changes based on their own knowledge, skills, and lived experience of the issues they encounter in their own lives. They recognize that positive health and well-being outcomes will not be achieved by the imposition of a top-down, "doing to" culture, and recognize that meaningful social change will only occur when people have the opportunities and resources to control and manage their own futures, and to find meaning and a sense of coherence in their lives.

Box 6 gives an overview of the C2 Connecting Communities program, which draws on assets approaches and complexity theory to rebalance power relations so that residents and service providers can work together to jointly problem solve and improve local conditions for well-being.

As the example in Box 6 demonstrates, localized and assets-based thinking is vitally important in helping to redefine relationships between citizens and service providers. Making this mainstream is more challenging, since it requires the buy-in of additional actors, such as the state and other key decision-makers. However, significant progress in thinking around well-being and the co-production of positive change across all levels of administration can be seen within the context of Scotland (United Kingdom). Widely known for its poor rates of morbidity and mortality, Scotland has set a progressive

---

* A focus on factors that support human health and well-being and emphasize the assets held by people and communities, rather than a focus on deficits and the factors that cause disease.

Box 6 **Creating a Collective Narrative—C2 Connecting Communities**

"It's not smoking, alcohol, obesity, or substance misuse which are the greatest determinants of poor health in low-income communities, but rather powerlessness, hopelessness, disconnectedness, and passivity. The former are merely ways of coping with the latter, with catastrophic health consequences."

—Hazel Stuteley, founder of C2, 2014

C2 is a community engagement program that has been transforming the health and social status of low-income communities in the United Kingdom since 1995. Through a process of community "health creation," C2 works by releasing the latent strengths of residents and service providers to work together as equals to jointly identify and solve problems and improve local conditions for well-being. C2 centers on establishing a long-term creative problem-solving partnership between residents and front-line services both from health and other agencies, e.g., housing providers, social services, local authorities, police, and fire services.

This involves working with residents and service providers to identify the multiple dimensions of the "problem space" (i.e., the historical, sociocultural, and economic factors) that have led to the "locked-in behaviors" of both staff and residents that create and perpetuate a deficit-based narrative and keep community health and well-being low. Through the development or reformulation of relationships based on respectful dialogue, trust, and humility, an enabling environment is created to release "opportunity spaces" in which the community and those working with it can self-organize to create a more positive environment and begin to create a new narrative based in strengths and agency. Although residents lead the partnership, it generates parallel action and learning among agency staff.

One example of a C2 self-organizing community can be seen in Camborne, Cornwall, United Kingdom, an area of high deprivation. The TR14ers dance group was founded jointly by young people and the local police force in response to local concerns around high levels of antisocial behavior and health inequalities among the town's young people. At the time, a narrative of shame and low self-esteem was prevalent among young people who felt stigmatized because of the poor reputation of their town. Indeed, the group named themselves after their postcode so that they could avoid using the word Camborne in their name.

In its first ten years, over 1,000 young people took part in the dance workshops. The town recorded the following measurable outcomes linked to the creation of the dance group: A 46 percent reduction in anti-social behavior; a 60 percent drop in the use of tobacco, alcohol, and other drugs; a 75 percent reduction in teenage self harm; a 22 percent increase in levels of educational attainment; a 90 percent reduction in truancy rates; a 62 percent reduction in poor behavior in school each week; and eight young people prevented from entering the criminal justice system. Through this program, young people have been able to reclaim the narrative of their community—instead of feeling shame, young people have improved self-esteem, self-respect, and leadership skills. The wider community also now views them as good role models who improve the image and reputation of the town. Indeed, the group has gone on to win a number of regional and national awards, which further cement its achievements.

C2 has long recognized the power of peer learning between communities, and now facilitates a national network of self-organizing communities who can share experiences and provide advice for other people wishing to transform local conditions and relationships with service providers.* [24]

path toward redefining relationships, cultures of working practice, and expectations around well-being from individual to governmental levels. In 2010, for example, National Health Service (NHS) Tayside launched its Health Equity Strategy: Communities in Control, to increase health and well-being and to foster community control in a way that gave people a meaningful sense of purpose and coherence in their lives. At the heart of this strategy was a commitment for the NHS to promote health as much as it cares for ill health; to work across the life-course; and to work jointly with communities, local authorities, and the voluntary sector in order to achieve this. Bolstered by other Scottish government–backed initiatives, the movement toward collaboration and shared problem-solving has gained traction in recent years, as can be evidenced in the establishment of ongoing and linked ventures, such as the Scottish Community Development Centre, the Scottish Co-Production Network, and the Communities Channel Scotland.†

* For more information and other examples of C2 and C2-inspired activities, see *www .c2connectingcommunities.co.uk*; *http://msaphase.org*

† For more information about these organizations, see the websites for the Scottish Community Development Centre at *www.scdc.org.uk*, the Scottish Co-Production Network at *http:// coproductionscotland.org.uk*, and the Communities Channel Scotland at *www.communityscot.org.uk*

The Impact of Social Media on Narrative

The way that we communicate in the modern media landscape has of course greatly reshaped the way in which health and well-being-related behaviors and narratives are influenced, often bypassing traditional information and communication channels. When harnessed effectively, social media can facilitate community empowerment and action, with positive impact on well-being and well-being-related behaviors. The #MeToo campaign is an obvious example that is working to change embedded narratives around gender and sexual harassment and the wider socio-cultural context within which they play out. Although originating within the American film industry, #MeToo has since influenced sectors as diverse as medicine, politics, religion, the military, and the porn industry, and has trended in scores of countries across the world. Although the direct impacts of the campaign are not always easy to isolate, emphasizing the magnitude of sexual harassment has enabled people to come forward to share their experiences as part of a global narrative, potentially laying the foundations for a cultural shift in the way that sexual harassment is understood and responded to.

The advantages of these advances in communication—speed, access, informality, individual ownership, and control—can also represent potential threats to the way a narrative is shaped. Misinformation and sensationalism, lobbying by industry, as well as fake news can generate falsehoods and distrust. Furthermore, when the narratives being pushed out exhort people to achieve, excel, be happy, and be positive, expectations are raised, with high levels of pressure placed on individuals to improve their situation rather than pointing to the need for societal-level policies and other actions. We are already seeing the downsides of this, with an accumulation of research now pointing to rising stress, anxiety, and other mental health problems, particularly among young people.

Establishing Accountability for Well-Being Actions and Narratives

While asset-based approaches have much to offer to culturally-relevant understandings of well-being, it is vital that they are not used to distract from wider debates around structural inequalities, and do not become a justification to defer responsibility for change solely to individuals and communities. Indeed, establishing where responsibility for well-being lies is a deeply contentious area, particularly where well-being is understood through diverse cultural narratives. Although a level of responsibility of course lies with the individual, it is also necessary for government and other key decision-makers to facilitate this through

---

Box 7 **Accountability**

The Right to Information (RTI) movement began in India in the 1990s against a background of endemic corruption in government services and in the provisioning of social entitlement. This movement recognized that a key obstacle to well-being at a local level was the lack of information available to people on their entitlements. In 1994, RTI organized public hearings—*jan sunwais*—to audit local-level development projects and payments, requiring all copies of documents relating to these works to be made public. Local government officials were not initially co-operative. However, as increasing numbers of people across the state began to hear the many stories of corruption that were emerging, they became empowered to act on this information. The hearings exposed the vast gaps between official project expenditure reported and actual expenditure, and led to nonviolent civic actions, boycotts, and sit-ins at government offices that forced those in power to become more accountable. Today, *jan sunwais* exist across large parts of India, and have become embedded as important enabling environments for the voices of marginalized communities to be heard, and for those in powerful positions to be held to account.[18,25]

---

the provision of the material and structural resources needed to enable this option to become feasible (see Box 7).

However, responsibility also critically depends on change from those who have the power to set the well-being agenda and narrative—the food, alcohol, tobacco, technology, "wellness," and pharmaceutical industries, for example, who too often remain complicit in keeping populations unhealthy, and whose actions are often overlooked, or even supported, by political agendas and the popular media. Important questions arise therefore over how to harness the compassion and co-operation of this wide diversity of parties and agendas so that all are working toward the common good, and all can be held accountable for their actions.

Learning to Listen

Many of the approaches outlined above share a central requirement, namely that those wishing to unpack well-being narratives first begin with listening to the communities or individuals whose well-being they are purportedly interested in. This is no small feat. Listening deeply and intently takes time and humility, neither of which are always available in abundance in academic research environments or national statistics offices, or neatly fit the political calendar or media cycle. Quantitative work on subjective well-being in particular is limited in the way it can respond and adapt to the rich nuances of well-being narratives. While it has to be reiterated that the quantitative work in this area has been of great value, it has come at the expense of the kind of embedded, participatory, subject-led research that this paper has outlined. Finding a way to evoke and capture, at scale, the well-being narratives of the grass roots seems an important step if we aim to make a convincing case for taking well-being seriously. An example of an initiative which has done this very well with regard to health (if not so much well-being) is Healthtalk.org, a website that provides free, high-quality information about health issues by sharing the lived experience of patients and caregivers. A resource such as this for individual and collective well-being narratives, one that allows qualitative researchers to really listen to what being well (or not being well) means in a given context, might actually help us interrogate "what makes life worthwhile."

If we are going to see a real shift in how governments and cultures define progress, we will need to shift to a well-being narrative that authentically expresses the nuances, cultural contexts, and lived experiences of people and communities, and that creates space and demand for solution sets and changes in expectations that advance well-being.

The Power of Shifting Narratives, Expectations, and Consciousness

Discussion and Case Studies From Bellagio

The late writer David Foster Wallace once addressed an audience of fresh college graduates with this parable:

> *There are these two young fish swimming along, and they happen to meet an older fish swimming the other way, who nods at them and says, "Morning, boys. How's the water?" And the two young fish swim on for a bit, and then eventually one of them looks over at the other and goes, "What the hell is water?"*[1]

The point, Wallace continued, is that "the most obvious, important realities are often the ones that are hardest to see and talk about."

Narratives—collections of stories that work together as a system to convey an interpretation of the world and how it works—are like Wallace's water: ubiquitous, consequential, and often subconscious. Narratives are expressed through cultural products,[2] such as language and storytelling, visual art and literature, news and entertainment media, commercial advertising, and political messaging. When expressed repeatedly, narratives also play a role in shaping culture[3] by establishing and reinforcing social norms and expectations.

Narrative was far from subconscious at Bellagio. It stood front and center, weaving through every topic of conversation from equity and grassroots engagement to cultural context, measurement, and political will. The common thread was a sense that narrative matters greatly, for its ability to reflect, reinforce, and change social norms, and that there is tremendous opportunity to shift from an economic-focused narrative about progress to one focused on well-being. Imagine the difference in attitudes, expectations, behaviors, resource allocations, and decisions if the narrative "what we value most and use as our sign of progress is consumption, wealth, and a strong economy," changed to "what we value most and use as our sign of progress is equitable well-being." Many of the practitioners who shared case studies at Bellagio are focused on narrative change as their leading or supporting strategy, and the social entrepreneurs in the group shared extensive insights on opportunities, challenges, and best practices for changing narratives.

Narrative Definitions

Just as multiple stories form a narrative, multiple related narratives often reflect a **meta-narrative**—an overarching (or underlying) storyline that connects the stories and narratives to a fundamental social concept, such as identity, community,[3] or well-being.

Narratives also play a role in creating and perpetuating prevailing notions of who should hold power and how power should be used, especially when they are determined and reinforced by the attitudes, beliefs, and values held by people in positions of power within a given culture, system, or social structure.

Narrative change aims to change the world—often by shifting power—at an ambitious scale by changing attitudes, beliefs, mindsets, and behaviors at the individual and community level, and by changing dominant narratives and often the policies and practices they advantage at the societal level.[3,4]

Why Narrative Matters

Narratives operate at an emotional as well as cognitive level. They can emerge organically, in response to the accumulation of similar stories and experiences, or they can be intentionally created as a tool for social change or oppression. Dominant narratives reflect the prevailing social and political assumptions about what is most expected, valuable, or desirable and, therefore, worthy of investment and effort. For example, Bellagio participant Kee-Seng Chia, founding dean of the National University of Singapore's School of Public Health, said that Singapore's rampant economic development over the past 50 years supported a narrative in which "wealth equals success, and you pursue wealth almost at the expense of everything else . . . even at the expense of health." The mindset that wealth is more important than health contributed to Singapore's "epidemic" of noncommunicable diseases, such as diabetes, Chia says, because people did not place a priority on developing habits and skills to create both wealth and health and then use those skills to achieve "resilience in both wealth and health."

Narratives don't just reflect assumptions, however—they also reinforce them. By telling people what to care about, narratives drive assessments of good and bad, right and wrong, success and failure. The dominant narrative about progress, for instance, determines what people measure to assess progress, and what policies and decisions they make to advance it. Narratives, as much as actual values or cultural contexts, drive how the media cover issues and what topics social "influencers" choose to address. Narratives also influence what policies and programs are implemented by power holders. For instance, if the dominant narrative defines social progress solely in economic terms, politicians and economists who are working to grow the economy have no incentive to change their tactics or to consider consequences to equity, the environment, or other factors, because according to the narrative, they *are* pursuing the outcome of greatest value. And, as we see when we look more closely at the current dominant narrative, this shapes not only societal attitudes, expectations, and priorities, but also individual choices and self-identity.

Critiquing the Dominant Narrative

As this book has explored, the dominant narrative on progress, in many places, focuses almost exclusively on economic factors, underscored by reliance on measures such as gross domestic product. Across most of the world, the message is clear: Wealth and consumption are the ultimate goal for nations as well as individuals, and therefore, are used to assess progress and power.

This narrative is not an objective truth, however. Like all narratives, it is based on an acceptance of assumptions built over time and molded and reinforced by current systems. And while economic indicators are sometimes held out as a proxy for how people and societies are doing, the existing dominant system and narrative certainly have not produced widespread well-being. In fact, as we have seen throughout this book, and as Chia's example above underscores, their impact on social attitudes and priorities has led to significant inequities and to deficits in health and well-being.

If the economic-focused narrative is so incomplete, should it be replaced with a narrative built around a framework of well-being, such as Bhutan's measures of Gross National Happiness? Not entirely, Bellagio participants advise. "Nobody, I hope, in a well-being space is saying that money and economy don't matter," says Liz Zeidler, chief executive of Happy City in the United Kingdom. "This sort of dichotomy just doesn't exist. Having enough money to get what you need in life, and more than that potentially, is an incredibly important part of well-being. It pays for many of the things that come with well-being. But it's not the end goal."

Rather than creating an either-or scenario, a more constructive approach would be to promote a narrative about progress that is centered on well-being *inclusive of* economic factors. "Instead of worrying about [economic factors] versus something else, [we should] sit down and model . . . how quickly developments would take place that would save money and build economic progress," suggests Bellagio participant Sir Harry Burns, professor of Global Public Health at the University of Strathclyde and Scotland's former chief medical officer.

Other participants, while agreeing that it's not a simple matter of privileging one narrative over another, see a need to explicitly confront the dominant narrative that economic success is an end in itself.

> *What we've got to do is really scrutinize: When is GDP useful? When is it not? In what circumstances does it have a place? But also recognize the huge number of perverse incentives . . . bound up in GDP.*
>
> —Katherine Trebeck
> Knowledge and Policy Lead
> Wellbeing Economy Alliance
> Scotland

Narrative's Role in Social Change

While dominant narratives often reflect and reinforce the status quo, narrative-change efforts aim to shift beliefs and behaviors in ways that change social policies, practices, power structures, and systems. Narrative change as a strategy can be used to advance more or less equitable worldviews, policies, and practices. Narrative change is also being used as a strategy for addressing social inequities because of the role narrative plays in perpetuating or contesting power dynamics. As Mallika Dutt, founder and director of the global initiative Inter-Connected, observed to Bellagio colleagues:

> *Inequities don't just exist because they exist. They exist because there are power dynamics that create power over structures, whether it's rich and poor, whether it's white and black, whether it's men and women, whether it's Indigenous and non-indigenous. . . . And it is usually when the people who don't have power in the traditional sense organize themselves that something shifts.*

Narrative change promotes social change first by questioning the underlying assumptions of the dominant narrative. Julia Kim, program director of the GNH Centre Bhutan, noted, for example, that social change agents might look at the pro-GDP narrative used by the United Nations to rank countries and ask: Who is actually happier, people in the develop*ing* country or the develop*ed* one? Using the term "developing," Kim says, creates an implicit assumption that a country, regardless of its cultural values and level of well-being, should aspire to one day be more like the "developed" country. Yet looking at the rising levels of stress, inequity, and overconsumption in many so-called developed countries, one might well ask whether some countries have in fact overshot the mark and become "overdeveloped." Next, narrative enables social change by offering a values-driven alternative that activates or challenges people's mindsets. To see how this works, one need look no further than the spectacular take-up of the narrative about income inequality, spawned in the first decade of this century by economists Thomas Piketty and Emmanuel Saez, among others.

How Well-Being Changes the Discourse

Economist Éloi Laurent, who teaches at Sciences Po Centre for Economic Research in France and at Stanford University, told Bellagio colleagues that he considers Piketty's income-inequality lens "the most successful strategy in shifting the debate from growth and GDP to well-being." In 2000, Piketty was a well-regarded rising economist but hardly a household name; he was mostly a wonk among wonks. But he was keenly attuned to capital, especially who holds it and how they use it. In 2001, he published *High Incomes in France in the 20th Century: Inequalities and Redistribution, 1901–1998,* which found that French income inequality had declined dramatically as the result of, among other things, the imposition of a state income tax.[5] More than 1,000 pages long and weighing over 4 pounds, some reviewers called the book "a door-stopping work of economic history."[6] But it succeeded in lifting up the topic of income distribution within public discourse.

Over the next five years, Piketty and fellow economist Emmanuel Saez published more on the topic, culminating in Piketty's book *Capital in the Twenty-First Century,* published in France in 2013 and in the United States in 2014. They were not the first publications to highlight changes in income inequality, but they fundamentally shifted the debate from one about trends in median income to one about gains at the very top of the income spectrum. Piketty's narrative, that "the consequences [of growing income inequality] for the long-term dynamics of the wealth distribution are potentially terrifying,"[7] captured the public imagination and inspired other writing and research.

Piketty's success in changing the analysis of income and, consequently, the conversation about wealth led to the use of new measures (focusing on top earners rather than median income), which prompted a new narrative (about income inequality), which fueled changes in political discourse and built movements (focused on addressing the unfair influence and gains of top earners), which led to social-change efforts that built currency for the new narrative. But how, specifically, does a *well-being* frame serve as a strategy for shifting the broader narrative about what individuals, organizations, communities, states, and nations should think and do?

The well-being narrative challenges a zero-sum mindset by promoting a more relational interpretation of the world. Unlike the distribution of financial resources, when well-being increases for some, everyone benefits, according to some economists who argue that an increase in well-being for one person or group does not necessarily mean a decrease in well-being for others. In fact, Harvard Medical School professor and researcher Nicholas Christakis has found that people's happiness depends on the happiness of others with whom they are connected, and in that sense, happiness is "contagious,"[8] notes Bellagio participant Karabi Acharya, director of Global Ideas for U.S. Solutions at the Robert Wood Johnson Foundation.

The well-being narrative gives decision-makers a new "north star" that is socially and morally conscious. A well-being frame broadens the narrative from a purely economic argument to one that has "moral heft," as Bellagio participant Jennifer Prah Ruger, Amartya Sen professor of health equity, economics and policy at the University of Pennsylvania, put it, because it introduces notions of justice and inequity. Similarly, shifting the discourse from "what we have to lose" financially to "what we have to gain" in terms of well-being has the potential to move society from a state of declining trust to a state of greater social cohesion and a sense of collective belonging and accountability. This is the theory behind the work of Bellagio participant Shariha Khalid Erichsen, managing partner of global investment and impact advisory firm Mission & Co., to help leaders of social-change organizations absorb the narrative, "well-being inspires well-doing." Erichsen's expectation is that the leaders' embrace of a well-being narrative will improve the well-being of their organizations, which in turn will lead to greater well-being in their communities.

The well-being narrative helps people envision a framework for change.

Social change involves two things: changing attitudes and changing behaviors. But the first step is to create meaning.

—*Éloi Laurent*
Senior Economist
Sciences Po Centre for Economic Research
France

And meaning can be hard to come by when issues are complex. Bellagio participant Danny Graham, CEO at Engage Nova Scotia, a coalition working to improve quality of life and economic conditions, knows this well. His challenge is to redefine what success means in a country with "abundant natural beauty, a strong sense of community belonging, and high life satisfaction," but a narrative that historically focused on sluggish economic and demographic growth. "The story we've been told and we've come to believe about ourselves is that our success should be measured by how fast we grow the economy," Graham said. "So, dating back to the 1930s, our province has been [issuing] reports [by] experts that ask and answer the question, what is the problem with us?"

Consequently, the average Nova Scotian equates employment with happiness, while the well-being movement operates in the margins of public consciousness. Graham's work seeks to shift the narrative to one that is based in Nova Scotia's intrinsic and culturally resonant community assets.

To test that approach, Danny Graham and his colleagues created a short video that highlights the province's assets rather than deficits and invites all Nova Scotians to join the conversation. "Here in Nova Scotia, quality of life is a point of pride," the video's narrator states:[9]

> *We are surrounded by beauty. We take time to have fun, and we care about how neighbors are doing. Those are the things that matter, we say. Success is about more than just dollars and cents. It's about how we look after each other, whether the air we breathe is clean, and knowing that kids . . . have a future. What if we all measured and paid attention to that bigger picture of what we value? Would we make better decisions? Would fewer people get left behind? Might we find new ways to work together? We think those are questions worth asking. What do you think?*

As examples like these illustrate, the effort to frame narratives around well-being is beginning to gain traction in fields like economics, in research institutions, and on the street. Now, how can that traction turn into a new dominant narrative?

Potential Strategies for Changing Narratives, as Raised at Bellagio

1. Lift up a simple, clear argument

Be clear about what you seek to change, how much, and by when. "Unless you articulate in quite some detail what it is you want to do, you just keep going around in circles," Burns states. Bellagio participant Tim Ng, deputy secretary and chief economic adviser of the New Zealand Treasury, elaborates: "[It] matters quite a bit who we're telling the narrative to, and what we're wanting them to do with the narrative, [because it affects] what we see as the vectors of change. If it is about shifting the social construction of values toward things we would [prefer] . . . then what we're trying to do is shift the political context and get people to better articulate what it is that they want from their governments."

Create a galvanizing statement that describes the desired change with consistent and repeatable resonance. In Bellagio, Zeidler called these "what-matters-to-us" statements—declarations that inspire people to respond, "Wow, that's a different way of looking at the future; let's organize around that." A good example comes from Scotland, Zeidler observed, where the statement *We want Scotland to be the best place for children to grow up* is embedded in the government's website, national performance framework, and countless forms of communication.[10]

One of the strengths of a narrative that emphasizes well-being is that people can relate personally to the message, which helps to make it galvanizing. But there are risks, too. A statement that resonates widely can be co-opted or pulled into so many other contexts that it changes or gets diluted. A statement that isn't clear and consistent can end up mobilizing people on behalf of the dominant narrative (e.g., if we improve well-being and reduce stress in the workforce, employees will be more productive); so can statements that try to monetize well-being, link it to extrinsic motivations, or focus on short-term gains. And even when the narrative is clear, consistent, and resonant, it isn't easy to move people toward change. Danny Graham recalls the excitement he felt when authors of Nova Scotia's decennial economic and demographic report agreed to highlight some of the cultural changes needed to make the country more "successful," including a suggestion by Graham's organization that economic growth should not be a proxy for more general success. By the time the report was published, however, the alternate theme had been edited out. Although the authors were open to the notion of well-being, they couldn't find a place for it within the traditional storyline, Graham concludes.

Hold a mirror up to underlying beliefs, assumptions, and knowledge. Lifting up the factors that either propel or impede progress, and engaging communities in articulating and defining what matters to them, makes the argument for change easier to envision. Bellagio participant Anita Chandra, vice president and director for RAND Social and Economic Well-Being, observed that hope and assets are more than the absence of deficits. A more effective narrative about well-being would talk about "the kinds of future states we want to get to" and capture assumptions about the "core elements of thriving," Chandra said.

2. Anchor the narrative in shared values

Social change experts agree on the importance of basing narrative on values, because values trigger beliefs and motivate behaviors. (*Whose* shared values? We'll get to that in a moment.) On the surface, the task of identifying shared values in an America deeply divided by politics, let alone perspectives on health, seems daunting. Fortunately, as Trebeck noted in Bellagio, scholars have identified 10 basic universal values, which either can support or undermine subjective well-being.[11] These values are triggered in people all the time, both directly and indirectly. "Different spaces, different regimes, different contexts illuminate and encourage [respective values] to flourish," Trebeck explains. "[Values can be] activated by advertising, or even by how a question is asked, or by education, or by physical environment." Or, crucially, by narratives.

The shared value of human and ecological interdependence—what scholars call "universalism"[12]—is especially relevant to a narrative about well-being. Kim illustrated this for Bellagio colleagues with a story about driving the California coast during the 2018 wildfires, which scientists say were exacerbated by an increase in hot, dry weather caused by climate changes attributable to human actions.[13] Similar rising temperatures in the Himalayas are causing glacial ice to melt.[14] "The problem is that, no matter how much Bhutan is trying to do to preserve the environment, because of this interdependence [with the actions of people and governments outside Bhutan] they're at risk of the bursting of glacial lakes and flooding in the country. As one of our ministers said, 'We cannot be a GNH [Gross National Happiness] bubble in a GDP world.'"

Show how a well-being approach fits with shared values—and how an economic-only model does not. Values can serve as the tool to both *tell* why the status quo is problematic and *show* what can be gained from change. The "telling" part of this guidance, according to Bellagio participant and journalist David Bornstein, co-founder and CEO of Solutions Journalism Network in the United States, often involves "revealing the lies and the deceptions and the false promises that are baked into the current aspiration and materialism in our world, and the false gods that we can call out with storytelling." The "showing" part involves connecting the proposed solution to the aspects of well-being that people care most about.

Take care not to perpetuate problematic values, especially those that have caused structural inequities and oppression and those that undermine well-being. Values-based narratives for change can be tricky, because many flawed values are so deeply rooted in individual and collective consciousness that they sneak back into the new framing of the problem. When the human rights organization Breakthrough, which Dutt founded and led in a prior role, began working to end violence against women and girls in India, for example, leaders knew they had to achieve many incremental cultural changes, such as persuading men to wear condoms when having sex with their wives or to stop marrying off daughters at an early age. The campaign created for Breakthrough by Ogilvy, however, couched the narrative in terms of protecting women—a concept based on very patriarchal values in India. In the end, Dutt told Bellagio colleagues, "We made a decision organizationally that, even if the campaign allowed us to reach [our short-term objectives], we could not use the patriarchal value as the lever. Because . . . then what we were doing was continuing to reify the same structure that was creating the problem in the first place."

There is another angle to this challenge. Some values that harm selected populations—usually people of color—have been allowed to stand, largely unchallenged, until they begin to affect more "powerful" (usually white) populations. For example, in the United States, mortality from diseases of despair, which often accompanies economic inequity, has plagued communities of color for generations but has only recently begun rising among white Americans.[15] A tension is emerging, notes Chandra, as constituencies mobilize around a new narrative of health and well-being to address diseases of despair. While no one wants to see any group suffer, she says, there is a need to reconcile cultural narratives and policies that are now newly disadvantaging some people, but have been in place for many years to disadvantage others over generations.

Listen to the community to shape the narrative and message

A new well-being narrative must be built on the wisdom, stories, and cultural strengths of people and communities—and this requires the involvement of people whose lives are affected by the narrative. That's what the Happy City Initiative did in Bristol, in the United Kingdom. "Our first two to three years were spent in the heart of communities, in schools, prisons, shopping centers, businesses, community halls," said Bellagio participant Zeidler, "finding out from 'non-experts' what mattered to them, how they viewed and sorted and found well-being, what a thriving place looked like."

Similarly, members of Engage Nova Scotia are in deep listening mode to identify their narrative change strategy. When policymakers weren't ready to adopt a well-being frame, Danny Graham told the Bellagio group, he and his colleagues surveyed 1,000 people to ask how they should gauge success. "Eighty-one percent said improving our quality of life, [while] 68 percent said growing our economy," Graham recalls.

Be humble. Remember that people have been talking about and living out their beliefs on well-being for millennia, through ancient philosophies and Indigenous cultures. "We haven't invented this," Zeidler cautions. "We've got to be really careful that we're not trying to come up with an answer and [assuming] the world will be okay when everyone thinks like us—because that's exactly the problem with the old paradigm."

Create space and build power so that those who have been oppressed by the status quo and dominant narrative can craft their own narrative about well-being. Narrative-change efforts that are driven from the top down by people in privileged positions won't get very far, says Bellagio participant Walter Flores, executive director of the Center for the Study of Equity and Governance in Health Systems, based in Guatemala and working globally. But in countries with young democracies, where civil society may not historically have had power, and in the historically marginalized communities of older democracies, work will need to be done to ensure voices that have been structurally excluded have the agency and platform to define their narrative and to fully participate in shaping the broader narrative around well-being.

Draw on cultural identity and pride as levers of change. Pride in one's culture is an essential ingredient of social cohesion and hope, both of which are crucial for advancing a narrative of well-being. In Bhutan, for example, the cultural context for a common well-being narrative has been influenced by the Buddhist notion of a "Middle Path," based on avoiding extremes, living with moderation, and balancing both the material and intangible conditions for well-being (as reflected in the nine domains of GNH). These domains are regarded as being interdependent—a holistic view that does not privilege economic factors above others, but places them alongside a range of social and environmental concerns.

This discussion of natural capital has inspired deep philosophical debates about human-centered versus eco-centric perspectives. Natural capital, a framework designed by economists, can be defined as "the world's stocks of natural assets, which include geology, soil, air, water, and all living things."[16] The concept is controversial in that natural capital, like monetary resources, becomes a social and economic liability (as well as an ecological one) when badly managed.[16] Ng notes that Indigenous people tell a much more "relational and integrated story" about the connection between humans and the natural environment, compared with the more transactional narrative of eco-system services.

Be sensitive to the meaning of words, to avoid reinforcing flawed paradigms.

Words can either bring people together or divide; whether you're rallying around the idea of happiness or the idea of well-being, words can either be pulling people together or putting a wall up.

—Richard E. Besser
President and CEO
Robert Wood Johnson Foundation
United States

"Resilience" is one example, and "success" is another. Used primarily in the West, where it usually indicates advancement toward personal wealth, the word "success" is largely irrelevant in many other cultures. "Progress" may be a better term, but it infers a trajectory that may be more linear than that of a well-being approach. Many other words used to indicate positive movement also have monetary connotations, such as value, rich, profit, investment. Even the use of "health" and "well-being" has implications for narrative. Instead of using one or the other, Chia suggests, why not talk about a culture of health *and* well-being, which has the added benefit of making the concept easier for people to understand?

Words also convey meanings linked to race, class, and culture. The bottom line: There is more work to be done on framing the meta-narrative around well-being, and it must be done in ways that engage and listen to communities and respect cultural context.

Meet people where they are

Take time to understand what people think. It is difficult to change someone else's understanding of the world without first knowing what they believe and what you want them to believe differently. Moreover, simply expressing a narrative doesn't guarantee that others will believe, trust, and own it. Successful narrative change, said many in the conversation, requires building a movement, or a network of believers. Danny Graham breaks it down even further: "You can only move at the speed of trust. And you begin by going slow to go long. . . . Sink your roots in as deeply as you can."

> *Start by asking questions rather than declaring your truths.*
> —*Danny Graham*
> *CEO*
> *Engage Nova Scotia*
> *Canada*

Engage with the opposition to mitigate challenges. New narratives that impact the status quo inevitably attract opposition from powerful interests fighting to preserve the dominant narrative. Working proactively to align the two sets of values can mitigate the opposition and broaden support for a new narrative. Engage Nova Scotia has taken this tack by building a coalition from diverse sectors (e.g., environment and industry); avoiding "political hijacking" by seeking government's support but not its leadership, and by ensuring diverse political representation on the organization's board; meeting consistently with opposition leaders to describe the well-being effort; and refraining from having senior government officials make high-profile announcements about the work that could attract scrutiny. This strategy has attracted enough support from potential opponents that the coalition's work has lasted through several election cycles.

Capture and share real-world stories to support the new narrative

Once people are engaged, how can the well-being narrative connect in ways that are relevant and tangible and that demonstrate how well-being can lead to better outcomes? That's where storytelling comes in: stories in the news media, social media, advertising, movies, video games, literature, art, and popular culture. Stories about what well-being means and about what does and doesn't work to achieve well-being. Stories about how individuals, communities, and systems can be transformed by a focus on well-being. Stories can be persuasive, but they are also "subversive," according to Bellagio participant Claire Nelson, lead futurist of the Futures Forum in the United States and the Caribbean, both because they slip into the consciousness and because they "make it comfortable for the oppressed to be able to engage in the discourse."

Indigenous cultures that have an oral tradition have long used storytelling as a tool to push for change, notes Bellagio participant Romlie Mokak, CEO at the Lowitja Institute, a Djugun man and member of the Yawuru people of Australia. "The power of the story to start to think, to start to activate. . . . This is where change may happen," he says. Bhutan's well-being effort has borrowed a page from that history, using stories to start conversations about what matters—to hold up the social "mirror" mentioned earlier.

Bornstein, whose work is all about storytelling with a purpose, emphasized to the Bellagio convening that some stories will reinforce narratives while others go in one ear and out the other. "And then there are stories that really [are] able to dislodge people from fixed positions—from a motivated denial of global warming, for one example, or from very strongly held beliefs," Bornstein says. "There are special stories that actually work best with the people who are hardest to convince." Understanding what those stories are is a key to gathering support for a new narrative.

Combine stories with metrics to make them more powerful. Just as stories add meaning to quantifiable measures (see chapter 4), metrics enhance stories to produce narratives that are both grounded in data and emotionally compelling. Zeidler posed the challenge this way: "How can we connect up the metrics and the stories at the global, local, and regional levels so that we can both learn from each other but also start telling more powerful narrative stories, by [having] some better connections between the metrics at those different levels?"

Engage voices outside the traditional health and social sectors to shape and carry the narrative

Remember Thomas Piketty and his narrative-shifting findings on income inequality? Piketty is an economist, not a professional in the health or social sector. So are Sir Angus Deaton and Anne Case, the scholars who advanced understanding of diseases of despair, and Paul Krugman, who popularized their findings in a widely discussed *New York Times* opinion piece.[17] Those contributions by people outside the usual sectors were game changers for the discourse on health and well-being. As Chandra observes, "We knew the data in the U.S. long before [Deaton and Case]. All public health leaders had seen the Centers for Disease Control and Prevention data over years. But until it was put together in that way, outside of traditional health, it didn't propel the conversation and capture a level of concern or attention." Deliberate efforts to engage these voices—and, as Erichsen suggests, to lift up stories of what other sectors are doing to promote well-being—are an important part of the strategy for building a new narrative.

Protect the narrative from misrepresentation. Engaging other sectors carries some risk, because not everyone outside the health and social sectors thinks about well-being in the same way. For example, many conflate well-being with wellness, so many lifestyle brands market well-being as relaxation, stress relief, and mindfulness. And not everyone sees increased equity, sustainable and responsible use, and conservation of the natural world or other factors in well-being as beneficial goals—from industries that advocate for unsustainable resource extraction to economic interests that advocate for tax policies that increase wealth disparities. And, as is the case in many social movements, some people, industries, and interest groups may co-opt the term and claim they are advancing a well-being framework while advancing principles and actions that can weaken the movement's credibility. The best defense against these risks is to make the narrative as clear as possible and ensure it is developed through authentic community engagement and tied to values that make it difficult to co-opt.

Shift narratives and consciousness at the individual as well as system level

Historic practices, particularly in capitalist or industrialized cultures, have trained people to place personal gain ahead of societal well-being, and to put the wealth of their own state or nation before global equity and sustainability. Systems, structures, cultures, and dominant narratives reinforce and reward this mindset and the behaviors that follow. For a new narrative to gain currency, and for public demand and support for a well-being approach to increase, it is important to shift individual consciousness and individual definitions of progress. Shifting the focus from "me" to "we" is a profound undertaking, but the well-being narrative is a powerful tool for doing so. Building on shared values, the narrative connects people to each other, their environment, and the planet. The public will that results leads to greater expectations, demand, and incentives for actions that support well-being.

The storytelling strategy described earlier is one tactic for shifting individual consciousness; another is to deliberately prioritize key constituencies. That is what Singapore's planned Healthy Campus Initiative is designed to do. This pilot initiative, which will operate at two major universities, aims to focus on university students—the country's future leaders—to replace the "wealth first" mindset with a "health and wealth" mindset and to become its lifelong ambassadors.

3. Organize around the new narrative

As the Bellagio conversation illustrates, narratives are important for many reasons, including their ability to influence norms and beliefs, to inspire hope, and to serve as a rallying point for action. For example, simply publicizing the fact that India has 37 million more men than women, and that the disparity fosters gender-based discrimination, did not change how Indian women are treated, Dutt observed to colleagues. "It is the organizing that the women's movement has been doing that has led to some policy shifts," she explained. The same can be said of social changes achieved through the LGBTQ marriage equality, Black Lives Matter, and #MeToo movements: it takes disciplined organizing around a new narrative for change to occur, and these changes help build the power of the new narrative and advance additional changes.

Potential Impact of Narrative Shifts

What can potentially come out of a new narrative centered on well-being? Can it focus attention on solving the inequities and structural barriers, such as racism, that prevent so many people from experiencing well-being? Can it move cultures from a mindset of "how much" to one of "enough"? Can it shift individual consciousness and build a collective consciousness in which the success of "we" is the success of "me," and oppression and injustice to anyone is injustice to all? And will those shifts drive meaningful societal change?

Examples discussed at Bellagio suggest that a compelling narrative—one that positions "improving well-being" as a central goal, reflects cultural values and contexts, and is reinforced through strategic storytelling—has potential to support all of these changes. In Bhutan, the well-being framework is a guiding principle for policy and planning at the national level and is reflected across several sectors, including tourism, education, and environment, with emerging initiatives in business and civil society. In Nova Scotia, a diverse coalition of supporters and partners has formed around the well-being narrative; social-service agencies have begun to incorporate well-being data into their strategic planning, and the provincial government is articulating a need to address inequality. In Paraguay and New Zealand, the well-being framework is built into the budgeting process as a core driver for decisions. And in Singapore, the political narrative has expanded to a more inclusive definition of success.

These may be early wins, but they are important ones. The challenge still ahead is to move from an overall societal narrative in which economies "need to grow, whether or not they make us thrive"—as self-described "renegade economist"[18] Kate Raworth says—to "economies that make us thrive, whether or not they grow."[19]

LEARNING FROM OTHER MOVEMENTS AND THE NEED TO SHIFT POWER

Historical oppression, structural inequities, and systems that protect existing power dynamics often result in many people's experiences and perspectives being ignored. This is particularly true for those who are the most impacted by decisions, including Indigenous peoples, youth, people living with lower incomes, women, and many others. In order for a well-being approach to take root and to achieve its potential to drive transformative change, it must be co-created with respect for cultural context, owned by communities, and include a shift in a traditional power structure that engages a broader and more diverse set of leaders.

Section 2 discussed how the very measures used to define well-being must be shaped by the populations they aim to measure; section 3 detailed how an authentic well-being narrative must come from people at the grassroots level. This section follows that theme by exploring how engaging people, organizations, and communities as valued stakeholders creates the best opportunity to develop an authentic well-being framework and to hold decision-makers accountable. While the shift to a well-being approach must be broadly based and include formal leadership structures, governments at all levels, the academy, international bodies, and the business community, it cannot be top-down.

How this shift forms and moves varies tremendously across different settings. In most cases, it will likely require some combination of public sector policy actions, incremental change from within systems, radical activism from outside the system, and engagement and integration of grassroots and social movements across all of these levers for change. This power shift can be both a vital part of well-being efforts and an outcome of the process itself.

The group at Bellagio recognized both the need for authentic grassroots engagement and shifts in power dynamics to build and establish currency for a well-being approach and to transform how societies define progress. The group explored potential pathways to shift power, increase grassroots participation, and effectively advance well-being, along with some potential risks and cautionary notes.

In chapter 7, "How Well-Being Relates to Resilience and Other Frameworks for Social Change," Bellagio participant Anita Chandra, vice president and director for RAND Social and Economic Well-Being, discusses resilience—a field of study that is complementary and related to well-being—to inform how well-being approaches will evolve in policy and practice. The concept of resilience comes up in other sections, including the cautionary note—offered here, in chapter 3, and in the Palestine case study—that in marginalized communities it can be read as both a positive indicator of well-being and as a means of downplaying or adapting to oppression.

The conversation about authentic engagement of people and communities and the real challenges of developing an equitable approach within inequitable systems wove throughout the Bellagio meeting. It is summarized in chapter 8, "The Imperative for Community-Driven Approaches and Radical Inclusion: Discussion and Case Studies From Bellagio."

How Well-Being Relates
to Resilience and Other Frameworks
for Social Change

ANITA CHANDRA, DR PH, MPH
Vice President and Director,
RAND Social and Economic Well-Being
RAND Corporation, United States

As well-being research and practice take root globally, it is useful to consider progress in related and complementary fields, such as the resilience framework, which has also relied on social change components to make progress. The resilience framework can inform the evolution and implementation of well-being science in policy and practice. In addition to the resilience framework, other efforts in population health and environmental sustainability may offer useful insights.

Social change is often defined as some type of group or collective action to advance change of any sort. There are many possible directions of social change, some of which affirm well-being and some that are in direct contradiction to it. For the purposes of this chapter, however, we use the term social change to characterize change that results from a reorientation of definitions, approaches, and actors to address long-standing, complex problems from a well-being and social justice perspective.

The primary focus of this chapter is on the resilience framework because it shares some of the characteristics of well-being research and practice, such as being broad and interdisciplinary, conceptually multidimensional,[1] occasionally controversial in how it is operationalized and applied, and foundational to other population, community, and environmental outcomes. Further, resilience and well-being frameworks are unfolding in parallel ways, galvanized by interest from nonprofit, philanthropic, business, and government sectors in collaboration. Recent efforts to create a well-being-based economy mirror many of the discussions in resilience, which have focused on constructs like determining the resilience dividend and organizing resilience strategy for local government.[2,3]

Perhaps the most important parallel between the well-being and resilience frameworks is the active consideration and treatment of equity. While much is being discussed globally about equity, or the fair and just access to opportunity, the actual integration of equity-based thinking has not moved fast enough in research and policy frameworks to realize the benefits we need societally. The well-being and resilience frameworks each necessitate central treatment of issues of equity because it is not possible to achieve these outcomes without deeper examination of how factors that drive inequity remain structural and systemic barriers to fully realized social change. It is important to disentangle how equity influences each framework, how connections can be created across frameworks to more effectively reorient approaches, how actors work together to solve massive social ills, and how we ensure full agency for actors often excluded from decision-making. In short, the equity barriers in the well-being framework (e.g., historical and legacy issues that impede progress for some populations) are not dissimilar to equity barriers in the other frameworks that give rise to problems discussed later in this paper, including environmental injustice (sustainability), intergenerational health disparities (population health), or fragile community systems that cannot recover from disaster (resilience).

Resilience is often defined as the ability of a system (human, community, etc.) to withstand and adapt to adversity.[4] At the individual level of subjective well-being, many argue that resilience, or an individual's ability to respond to stress, is a central feature of positive well-being, along with dimensions such as optimism and hope.[5] Community resilience entails the ongoing and developing capacity of the community to account for its vulnerabilities and develop capabilities that aid that community in (1) preventing, withstanding, and mitigating the stress of an incident; (2) recovering in a way that restores the community to a state of self-sufficiency and at least the same level of functioning after an incident; and (3) using knowledge from a past response to strengthen the community's ability to withstand the next incident.[6]

Connections between resilience and well-being are not simply at the individual level. When researchers and policymakers consider the interaction of social and ecological systems, they are often intersecting elements of well-being and resilience.[7-10] That is, the production of human potential (well-being) in a group or community is tied to the dynamic changes in its natural, built, or physical environment (resilience). These changes can be a result of acute (e.g., natural disaster) and chronic stresses (e.g., community violence) that affect the quality of that environment. For instance, the Programme on

Ecosystem Change and Society (PECS), an initiative of the International Council of Science (ICSU), "aims to integrate research on the stewardship of social-ecological systems, the services they generate, and the relationship among natural capital, human well-being, livelihoods, inequality, and poverty."[11] The integrative agenda of PECS is representative of other global recognition and trends to ensure that choices and decisions about the future of populations and places on the planet are grounded in the appreciation of both resilience and well-being together.

Yet despite these types of social-ecological frameworks, there are limits in the connections being made at the policy, programmatic, and resource level between the concepts of resilience and well-being. *The fields continue to move mostly in parallel, in limited cases making substantive connections in policy and program development. This seems to be a missed opportunity for policy and resource alignment, for considerations of equity, and for reorientation to the relatively antiquated social systems that require some revisioning.* In addition to the opportunities from the interconnections with resilience concepts, we briefly discuss opportunities in social change revealed by other areas of population health and environmental sustainability, which are on similar trajectories and can offer lessons learned that can inform the well-being framework. In this chapter, we examine interconnections and insights from these broad-scale social changes, with a particular focus on these aims:

- To connect the interest in strengthening resilience with efforts to build and improve individual and community well-being.
- To briefly summarize other areas of broad social change that may inform the unfolding of well-being research and policy to effect change and improvement in community and national outcomes.
- To chart a potential path forward, and identify key questions facing the synergistic fields.

Why Connect Resilience and Well-Being Frameworks

Despite challenges such as identifying a single path or direction or balancing resilience investments, the resilience framework is a paradigm that will likely stay and gain currency for a few key reasons that cut across sectors and disciplines and are also applicable to the well-being framework. **First, a resilience framework values complex and multisectoral collaboration and coordination** in order to achieve the ultimate end of "bouncing back" or "bouncing forward."[12] The orientation to whole of government and whole of community response and alignment is *intrinsic* to the resilience framework. Thus, while we have increasing policy directives globally, nationally, and locally to foster new and often unique partnerships, resilience provides a framework for how to consider and evaluate those relationships and pull apart which organizations are truly response reliable, and which are not. This also comes at a time when we are not only expecting more from our partnerships, but more from our local leaders—to be open to what is unseen and assume both a creativity and humility in how options and decisions are developed and evaluated. But, there are significant policy questions governing the multisectoral coordination required to advance resilience thinking and conduct that cross-sectoral collaboration in an efficient manner and in consideration of community development.[13] These policy questions include: What are the right incentive structures to motivate this type of collaboration? What is the right risk-based or other type of governance structure? What are the ways to most effectively leverage the insights from each sector about assets, risks, and hazards, and integrate that information into a common operating picture to inform decision-making? How do we create resilience-based metrics for a shared accountability framework? Well-being frameworks, such as the one being used in Santa Monica, California, are working to link well-being measures to city performance management.[14]

Second, the resilience challenge for 21st-century cities requires data and emerging technologies (e.g., in the context of smart cities) to be integrated across seemingly disparate groups and sources *and* for those data to be transformed and translated into information and insight for immediate application.[15] In order to capture the most useful information on shocks and hazards; the ecological and social impacts of those stresses; and the pathways to response, mitigation, and adaptation, policies that govern data use and stewardship will be more profound. Data use and application is not new, but in an era of government 2.0,[16] government 3.0, web 3.0, and beyond—in which the range and types of data are more available to a broader set of citizen analysts and the expectations of accountability are heightened—resilience thinking about what is useful from traditional data on assets and risks becomes more important.[16] Will these data really provide insight on community capacity or capability, or does it lack that signal? Does a community have information that will facilitate decisions to enhance resilience? How should a city use new forms of data (e.g., from sensors, social media), and what policies will best support that use?

Third, resilience constructs require active consideration of the connection between people and place, between the activities that happen in social institutions and the physical conditions that surround them. Historically, those individuals who endeavored to address infrastructure resilience were separate from those who sought to address aspects of human resilience, health and well-being, or psychological resilience. But now, particularly in the context of city planning and response, there is clearer understanding that these disciplines must work in concert and be represented in more cohesive policies that braid the human and infrastructure or environmental aspects of resilience. The policy challenge is how to create that *transdisciplinary* lens to policy and have those perspectives carry through in all city programs, funding, and other resource planning.[17] Further, there are questions on how best to craft policy that can simultaneously address issues from the environmental impact of demographic or social stresses, along with the resulting effects on social cohesion or community organization. In this context, there are also questions about where resilience-based investments will be most impactful and what the social and economic returns on investment (ROI) are. To date, policy frameworks and approaches to policy analysis have struggled with this integrated approach and consideration of investment.

Finally, resilience thinking comes at a time when the views of government and the role of the private sector are fundamentally shifting. There is a stronger focus on public-private partnership, but what constitutes public-private benefit, and what is needed in the coordination among a wide variety of private sector entities—business, nonprofit, and so forth—remains a question. Understanding the roles and purpose of civil society organizations in gathering information and responding to shocks and stresses also remains unclear.[18] These civil society organizations can be key leads for addressing issues of equity, community affordability and livability, and social protection, but to date, often lag behind in their representation in policy. Questions abound regarding how to better engage these organizations and what are the civil society policies that are most coherent and effective for promoting resilience.

Resilience and Well-Being: Lessons Learned

This context for the resilience framework and connections to the well-being framework are not simply revealed in the decisions ahead, but also in the motivations for why resilience emerged as important. Further, the complexity of resilience thinking has challenged fields to come together, as is also true with a well-being approach.

Why has resilience thinking become this important, and what does it motivate in community organizing and planning?

The increasing rate of disaster begs the question whether national or global plans, capacities, or resources will be effective in addressing the mounting economic, ecological, health, and social costs of disasters, particularly in the context of other community stressors, such as poverty and violence.[19] The last decade has marked increasing focus on the resilience of people and places—in brief, how well do society and our institutions confront a set of risks, stresses, and disasters, and why do some populations or certain communities handle those challenges more effectively? While a seemingly straightforward question, the solution set to make all populations and communities more resilient is not simple. There are significant issues regarding how populations and communities assemble and make decisions to build resilience in ways that are equitable.[20] Further, a solution set has not been easily translated into commonly accepted resilience policies, a final and robust set of resilience metrics, or a single blueprint for resilience action.[21,22] Despite some continued fuzziness in the field and the lack of a resolution around those policies and action steps, the resilience framework continues to be reflected in national and global strategy, local policy, and the research agendas of a range of academic and policy institutions. Why? And through this lens of resilience, what can we learn from related fields of well-being that might advance future synergistic actions between the two?

The resilience framework has assumed new resonance in global dialogue about chronic stress and the well-being of populations, increasing inequities and income inequality, significant demographic transitions, and changes in global climate. This complex backdrop and interplay of multiple challenges has made community resilience not only the *term du jour*, but has highlighted resilience as a necessary pathway to the future viability of populations and the ability of social and physical structures to withstand and adapt to a wide variety of threats. In a single term, resilience and its associated derivatives—individual, community, systems resilience—has moved from a "nice to have" to an expected ability that every community needs in order to survive, thrive, and flourish.[23]

It is presumed that communities that do not attend to actively building resilience capacities and capabilities are destined to lack the wherewithal to address the complex set of challenges of the 21st century and beyond. Given this urgency, it is also important to understand how communities that do not automatically have the access to the formal structures and means to build those resilience capabilities and capacities can build grassroots movements to counter those challenges in ways that do not place them further at risk.[24] On the other hand, building community resilience can be a path to addressing power structures and motivating local change,[25] such as through ideas like building the urban green commons[26] or grassroots localization.[27]

Connecting resilience, science, and practice across disciplines and sectors can be difficult, as it is for well-being approaches.

The field of resilience has mostly evolved in parallel until recent years. Social scientists and natural scientists have often worked in separate streams, with limited connection and alignment. For example, psychologists have profoundly deepened our understanding about how exposure to childhood traumas can not only influence the formative periods of childhood development, but can shape lifespan trajectories and create conditions for success or less positive outcomes later in life.[5,28] Sociologists have explored aspects of resilience, with particular attention to neighborhood structures, social cohesion, and other aspects of social organization. Political scientists and other policy experts have examined the governance structures that promote adaptive capacity at municipal and federal levels.[29] Economists have only begun to capture the benefits of resilience and whether certain types of strategies can yield value on a community's adaptive capacity.[2] On the natural science side, the forces of climate and environmental impacts have propelled the field, particularly informing best approaches to mitigation and adaptation, ways to construct green and resilient infrastructure, and strategies to finance investments in the ecosystem that will confer resilience benefits.[30] These scientists have also raised up discussions of the intersection of weather-related events and other community stress, and how those factors interplay to put some communities at greater risk for disaster and longer and more arduous recovery periods. These disciplines have built on a long history of systems-dynamics thinking that has crossed the fields of mathematics, physics, and operations research, to name a few.

Community resilience attempts to bring the disciplinary elements together by building on the interaction of natural, physical, financial, human, and social capital,[31,32] all drivers of resilience capability. Social capital is enhanced by participatory decision-making and partnerships between government and nongovernmental organizations.[6] Communities with robust social networks often have a greater ability to coordinate disaster recovery, and as such, the interaction among human and social capital is key to resilience.[33,34] All of these efforts to connect are valuable, but the challenge of creating transdisciplinary frameworks and integrated change are easier to articulate rather than implement given difficulties in current government and governance structures that can reinforce siloes and misalign incentives.

While the field is now challenged by how to bring together the disciplinary threads briefly summarized above, difficulties also remain in the practical applications of resilience concepts. New government initiatives, research investments, and philanthropic programs have emerged dedicated solely to supporting cities to develop resilience capacities and capabilities with particular attention to the ecological, economic, social, and broader public health consequences. Some of the key challenges that communities face in implementation of the resilience framework are likely to be instructive for well-being approaches, particularly for community well-being. There are some tensions in clearly capturing the cultural and contextual factors that can inform resilience, and some pushback on the term resilience as undermining discussions of equity and promotion of the idea of "equitable resilience" that takes into account access to power and resources.[35] For instance, some community groups have expressed concern that in implementation, resilience might provide an "out" to government leaders to put the burden of disaster recovery on community residents.[36] This is an important consideration regarding how broad social changes like resilience must not gloss over structural and long-standing issues, but rather provide an opportunity to highlight issues that have not been put together to demonstrate interconnections between resilience and equity, or resilience and structural racism, for example.

What are paths ahead for considering resilience and well-being frameworks together?

This context of resilience raises several opportunities and key practical questions that will confront the diverse sectors that also drive community functioning and overall community well-being. These include how to translate resilience science into the development of whole-city resilience strategy; building resilience capacity and testing that ability; working with vulnerable populations to improve resilience in ways that are equitable; or creating climate adaptation and mitigation plans that deal with a range of impacts, whether from episodic disaster or long-standing environmental degradation (e.g., work across global contexts to address issues of land use and loss, water policy, and other environmental consequences). Further, there are few methods to value investments in resilience frameworks.[2] As more communities begin investing in resilience frameworks, there is a growing need to improve approaches that can handle cross-sector lessons on resilience and convey the benefits of resilience-building investments. For example, there are developing methods to assess the extent to which green infrastructure choices mitigate the health impacts of climate change and to use insurance models to incentivize businesses to employ resilience-based plans in order to shift the probabilities of future damages from stochastic shocks (i.e., natural and manmade disasters, climate change).[37] There is some work evaluating singularly focused resilience interventions,[38] but little that places a relative value on resilience-specific benefits. When community leaders make choices about where to invest, it is essential that they have a sense that the investment will lead to resilience outputs and outcomes for both human and infrastructure benefit. This opportunity to examine co-benefits of resilience-based choices, such as the impacts on equity, human health benefits, and environmental equity, can also increase well-being. As such, resilience investment planning is also well-being investment planning.

Brief Overview of Key Insights From Other
Social Movements for Well-Being

While the resilience framework offers one of the better connections to well-being approaches as explained earlier, there are important insights from other fields of population health and environmental sustainability, both fields that have been propelled by broad social change and may prove useful for the well-being framework. We briefly cover those insights in this section.

Brown and Fee (2014) described the role of social movements in advancing population health, most notably linking social change and political mobilization as central to improving urban conditions and supporting the health and well-being of children.[39] The authors describe how outrage and concern about housing conditions, hygiene and sanitation, and environmental exposures galvanized improvements for health outcomes and energized political and civil society leaders to promote health. In the area of children's health, concerns about working conditions and youth labor, as well as the rise in the recognition of child maltreatment, had cascading impacts on child health outcomes. In both of these examples, broad-scale social change for population health was first ignited by a relatively bounded concern (e.g., housing), and then that focus helped to unpack the multidimensionality of the issue. Much like resilience has roots in concerns about acute disaster response, but then expanded to consider broader community stress, social change that actively moved the needle on population health outcomes often had this same trajectory.

Health in all policies (HiAP), a centering framework now in population health that is grounded in the idea of cross-sectoral engagement in all health practice and decisions, also offers a transferable model for well-being approaches. Shankardass (2018) describes the implementation challenges of a HiAP framework for sustained government practice, arguing the need for a leadership framework that links actions and incentives within and across sectors to ensure there is both consistent narrative leadership and financial alignment to achieve intended health outcomes at a systems level.[40] These insights about leadership and governance structure from HiAP raise questions for the well-being framework in terms of how to create the right structural map for sustained integration and accountability to a common set of well-being expectations and outcomes. Well-being faces similar concerns in how it is being integrated into existing decision-making structures.

In addition to these structural changes that led or have been leading to broader improvements in population health, there is an element of population health change that requires grassroots and advocacy-based strategy. For example, Hoffman (2003) examines why health reform approaches that have typified other social change in the United States did not originally coalesce into an effective strategy to advance universal health care coverage but started more narrowly on single health issues affecting particular groups.[41] She argues that it is the increasing engagement of grassroots voices that has been turning the orientation from narrowly focused, single-issue health movements toward a broad-scale change agenda, such as that which is focused on an interconnecting platform, such as universal health care reform. In the United Kingdom, the People's Health Movement includes an assumption that public health researchers will engage more in advocacy and political mobilization as part of their duties. Kapilashrami (2016) argues that the challenges that public health professionals face in supporting more advocacy-based movements—in short, the tension between professional practice and personal passion—can be surmounted, and that any improvements in health outcomes and health equity specifically require public health professionals to now span the boundaries of science and advocacy.[42] While the point may be controversial, the underlying conceptualization that broad social change requires experts to engage in this way in health is an important insight that may inform whether and how well-being research is applied for long-term impact.[43] In short, how do researchers, practitioners, and advocates in well-being work together effectively if we are to realize true social change?

Another area that provides insight for the future of well-being research and practice is the long-standing area of environmental sustainability.* There is much that has been written about this field and the social change that surrounds it, but we briefly summarize two points here that may be relevant to well-being approaches. First, environmental change and sustainability has focused on the power that a broad-based agenda can have for behavior change. Barr (2013) described how market-based approaches for "sustainable lifestyles" have provided inroads into motivating individuals toward social good choices.[44] The authors describe the powerful role of social marketing to excite individuals to pursue sustainability-based actions, and the use of market segmentation to help communities and policy leaders link behavioral motivations to particular characteristics of subpopulations. This insight about the role of behavior change around lifestyle adoption in sustainable

---

* There are many definitions of environmental sustainability. We use this one here: "Sustainability is the ability to meet the needs of the current generation without compromising the ability of future generations to meet their needs. The environment is the primary but not the only consideration within sustainability; it is important to also consider human welfare. Therefore, a sustainable society is one that protects natural resources while ensuring social justice and economic wellbeing for all" (University of Maryland Office of Sustainability, *https://sustainability.umd.edu/how-would-you-define-environmental-sustainability*).

practice has potential resonance in something as multidimensional as well-being. Similar marketing approaches may be compelling to advance lifestyle adoption around well-being.

The other component of environmental sustainability that may have application to the well-being framework is the expansion of sustainability to include social and economic constructs, such as human dignity and equity. The expansion to concepts like social sustainability has allowed environmentalists to look at the effects of environmental action on economic and social outcomes and vice versa.[45] Hawkins (2010) describes how a field like social work, traditionally focused on social systems and the welfare of people, is increasingly considering the role of the physical environment and environmental justice.[46] Business leaders are increasingly making the shareholder and bottom-line economic case for linking social and economic outcomes with environmentally sustainable practice.[47] In each of these examples, environmental sustainability has motivated social change through a broader lens that connects dimensions, a similar opportunity for well-being approaches.

Key Components of Well-Being and Linkages to Resilience and Other Broad Social Changes

The progression of the resilience framework—from definition to conceptualization to local action—provides a useful roadmap for discussions about well-being measurement and policy, and provides context about the connections between what has motivated resilience thinking and what has propelled global discussions of the well-being framework. Further, the discussion of the resilience framework and its core components offers a set of linkages to core dimensions of the well-being framework. In addition, the insights from social movements in population health and environmental sustainability offer perspective for the well-being framework as well.

Like resilience and other broad social concepts, well-being is defined with both subjective and objective assessment, and includes individual and community-level measurement.
Well-being comprises both individual and community dimensions. Individual well-being can be defined as the extent to which people experience happiness and satisfaction, and are realizing their full potential. When a person believes his or her life is going well and is functioning positively, he or she can be considered to have high levels of individual well-being. As noted earlier, individual resilience speaks to an individual's ability to withstand and adapt

to stress. As such, positive outlook contributes to that stress adaptation, but stress response also speaks to the kinds of competencies that are central to realizing full human potential (e.g., the ability to learn from challenge).

Community well-being is the collection of community status, features, and amenities that support or detract from well-being of individuals and community as a whole.[48] Key aspects of community well-being include community health, economic resilience, and educational capacity and environmental adaptation. In order to capture both individual and community well-being together, subjective (e.g., perceptions of the community) and objective (e.g., availability of resources) data should be included. In recent evolutions of community well-being, there is recognition of the role of *civic* well-being, or the governance, policies, and resources that embed supports for well-being in ways that are equitable. As noted earlier, environmental sustainability is multi-level and increasingly being linked to concepts like social sustainability. Its treatment of community investments and civic processes in areas like environmental governance offers perspective for well-being. For instance, environmental governance often examines environmental protection in the context of globalization and the development of market-based incentives.[49] Given the similarly cross-sector settings in which well-being, like environmental quality, is produced, it may be essential to consider how globalization or the interdependencies among actors and sectors can be exploited to promote well-being. Market-based incentives to promote movements like decarbonization or to value ecosystems can be assessed in the context of well-being. For instance, what is the market valuation of well-being?

Like resilience-based policy—as well as efforts in population health and environmental sustainability—putting well-being at the heart of policymaking is a new and promising approach at local and national levels.
Government implicitly wants to improve the well-being of its residents. But, due to political and administrative cycles, most governments tend to focus on short-term and intermediate milestones with the hope that this will eventually advance well-being. This type of approach can mean that policies miss the interconnections of investments to ultimately improve well-being. It can also mean that "patterns of well-being, over time, and within a geographical area are not fully understood."[50]

As resilience and sustainability frameworks have required more consideration of cross-systems thinking and multidimensionality (e.g., social and natural systems), measuring well-being, and understanding the determinants of well-being and how they interact, can help create a more holistic and informed policymaking approach.[51] Approaches for measuring well-being and quality of life are not new. However, the last decade has demonstrated how policymakers' use of well-being data to drive policy has gained real traction.[52,53] Several nations have included measures of subjective well-being in official dashboards, such as Canada, the United Kingdom, France, Italy, Australia, Chile, and many others. In addition, there are new movements to advance well-being in national and local doctrine and budgets. The city of Santa Monica, California,[14] now uses a well-being framework to inform local action and resource allocation, and countries such as New Zealand[54] have made news about their orientation to a well-being-based economy.

The well-being framework is now at a similar implementation stage as the resilience framework, with challenges in how to translate that information into meaningful action that can be executed by communities as a whole.
As fiscal resources become increasingly limited and there is more recognition of the breadth and diversity of actors in our communities, it has become more important for government and those organizations outside of government to help make communities healthy and well. But, there have been two challenges. First, most of those community initiatives have stopped short in strengthening well-being by focusing on some aspects of health, economic productivity, or wellness, with a less integrated focus on the roots of well-being, including the connections among residents and the organizations that support them to live full lives. Second, integration of a well-being framework at all levels—and as a lens and approach for all policy and practice—has not been completely achieved, and requires fundamental changes in how governments work (breaking silos, etc.). But the increasing imperative to reduce costs and increase positive outcomes can open space for approaches like well-being and resilience with the potential to demonstrate social, environmental, and economic ROI.

Well-being assessment, much like challenges facing resilience, holistic health, and sustainability policy, currently does not fully engage the range of government and nongovernmental organizations that contribute to well-being at the community level.
Government and nongovernmental organizations must work together to improve a community's well-being, a finding that also has been central to the field of community resilience, health in all policies, and sustainability. Communities that have strong integration of government and nongovernmental organizations are better able to support community response to any type of stress, given understanding of local assets and ability to mobilize resources at the right time and form.[28,55-57] From lived experience and insight into potential solutions to cultural context and Indigenous knowledge, engaging the grass roots and organizations tied to the community can help advance well-being solutions and approaches that would not otherwise be seen. Groups that are organized ahead of time

can play key roles in times of stress, and in an ongoing capacity, can strengthen overall well-being.

There are several elements of well-being that are also central to a community's ability to respond and recover from stress and degradation in resilience and sustainability theory. These are: economic vitality, social connection, community health, health equity, and the quality of context and place.

Economic vitality is essential to community well-being and can include indicators such as involuntary unemployment or productivity. A number of groups are vulnerable based on life circumstances (e.g., a lack of economic, cultural, or social resources), and these experiences can impede well-being.[7,28,58] When these populations are not reaping the benefits of economic resources and productivity, it becomes much more difficult for the entire community to develop and maintain resilience in the face of any stress.[28,59,60] In order to build and maintain well-being, communities must engage in equitable and inclusive economic development and reduce social and economic inequities. According to Pfefferbaum et al. (2009), resilience and, ultimately, community well-being depend on ongoing investments in physical resources, including schools, health facilities, job training, and neighborhood development.[60]

Social connections are an important dimension of well-being, yet were often overlooked in city planning efforts. However, increasingly, the issue of social connection and isolation is being understood by the public and private sector as a greater contributor to economic vitality and health outcomes (e.g., diseases of despair)[61,62] than perhaps previously appreciated. For many years, research has demonstrated that individuals who live in healthy and connected communities have better psychological, physical, and behavioral health[63] and are more concerned with maintaining their connections to the community over the long term.[64,65]

Community health also contributes to well-being, particularly aspects of emotional wellness, trust and belonging, and resilience and vitality. The underlying physical health of the population (e.g., prevalence of chronic conditions)[66] and psychological health[28,60] can greatly affect the community's well-being. While understanding the pre-existing health conditions of a community is critical for well-being assessment, it is also key to examine the historical stresses and strains that contribute to health inequity over time, such as community allostatic load.[67]

Finally, place can influence resident perceptions of their well-being and drive engagement in healthy behaviors, ultimately supporting a place to be more resilient. As noted earlier, socio-ecological frameworks purposefully intersect the realization of human potential and well-being with the ability of the environment to respond and adapt. Local context can include everything from green space availability to transportation options and efforts to address or adapt to climate change. Dimensions such as urban sprawl—a measure of the built environment that encompasses residential density, land use mix, centralization, and street connectivity (the degree to which destinations can be reached in a direct pathway)—have been linked to a variety of health and well-being outcomes. Further, urban sprawl and street connectivity are hypothesized to affect health outcomes through their effect on the opportunity for routine, daily physical activity. In concert with this hypothesis, earlier studies have shown that individuals in neighborhoods with a high degree of street connectivity walk and bicycle more.[68,69] Neighborhood safety and deterioration are also linked to poor well-being. Finally, communities that have plans to address a range of resilience-based challenges, such as changes in climate from rising sea levels to changes in precipitation (whether adaptation, such as floodplain management, or use of green or eco-approaches to construction), are often better equipped for changing demographic and economic conditions, and thus better able to withstand a range of stressors. Further, these communities tend to have individuals who view their local context more favorably.

Where to Go From Here: Opportunities for Linking Resilience, Health, Sustainability, and Well-Being

There are benefits in linking the resilience, sustainability, population health, and well-being discussions. First, the concepts are inextricably linked in both directions when considering the intersection of human potential with dynamic and changing environments. A resilient system is required to foster the best conditions for individual and community well-being; well-being assets in communities are an essential component of what makes an environment able to respond and recover from adversity. Further, the four fields uniquely capture the integration of multiple disciplines and sectors as a necessity and require whole-community planning.

Second, resilience, sustainability, holistic health, and well-being discussions have been motivated by common concerns. That is, that current plans for the 21st and even 22nd centuries fall short in harnessing individual and community assets and do not adequately consider how those assets interact with increasing challenges from multiple and overlapping stresses. This includes how we design government (e.g., do our usual government departments make sense if well-being, resilience, and sustainability are joint goals?); how we use technology to assess improvements in resilience and well-being performance and capacity (e.g., how should we use sensors, surveillance, and social media to flexibly assess these capabilities and outcomes?); and how we create incentives for conceptual, difficult objectives (e.g., what do we value and monetize for resilience and well-being?).

Third, these areas overlap in core capabilities. The well-being themes of outlook, agility, and flourishing are complementary to resilience themes of adaptation and response to adversity, holistic health themes around thriving, and environmental themes about ecosystem health and multi-generational sustainability. There remain questions about how well human potential is unlocked with and without adversity, but at the very least, capabilities such as fluid memory, appreciation of divergent thinking, creativity, and other aspects that we hold more central to meta-learning or 21st-century learning have a foundation in both well-being and resilience research at least.[70]

Finally, there are significant equity questions that cut across all of these fields, which require a deeper treatment of structural, historical, and intergenerational barriers to change.

As noted earlier, despite these linkages, the fields continue to move mostly in parallel. It is important to consider the key questions raised in this chapter around systems change, narrative development, transdisciplinarity, incentive alignment, and advocacy among others, and to identify ways to better sort within and across potentially aligned efforts for social change.

The Imperative for Community-Driven Approaches and Radical Inclusion

Discussion and Case Studies From Bellagio

To move the well-being framework from an aspiration to transformative action, it is imperative that people and communities are actively involved in both the conception of what it means and the implementation of this work on the ground. Too often, agendas for a "better world" have been top down, imposed by an elite few without truly engaging, listening to, and, importantly, ceding power to the people who both have untapped wisdom and who will benefit or be harmed by such approaches.

Much of the discussion at Bellagio centered on this crucial need for deep grassroots engagement and shifts in power, recognizing that this is not a conversation new or unique to the well-being movement, but one that has existed for decades across every social justice issue. With respect for the fields of community development and organizing, anthropology, and others who have developed countless theories, approaches, and tools to do this work, this chapter summarizes the conversation about how engagement and power shifting plays out differently in conversations about a well-being approach. When well-being is defined as people having what they need to thrive and pursue the future they want, deep engagement to understand what they actually want is inherent.

On its surface, the well-being framework sounds like something everyone can agree and aspire to. But for the notion of well-being to become real and tangible for all people it will require deeper, messier, and more systemic changes than its seemingly unobjectionable name first suggests. It will require a conscious effort to bring people from many and diverse communities to the table with real decision-making power, not as token representatives of a particular demographic group. It will require looking for ways to build power among people who have been oppressed, excluded, or denied participation.

Bellagio participant Walter Flores, executive director of the Center for the Study of Equality and Governance in Health Systems, based in Guatemala and working globally, called this "voice with teeth" and described it as a change in power dynamics that seeks to address structural and systemic oppression and advance equity. The promise of this approach is that it can ultimately lead to much more lasting change than a typical check-the-box consultation of the community approach. The well-being framework, with its emphasis on ongoing subjective inputs from all sectors of the community to define what well-being means and to measure progress, cannot succeed unless all groups are consulted, holding power, and helping to assess results.

> There is a difference between having a voice and having a voice with teeth, which means that you are the voice-active. So in voice with teeth, an authority is going to respect your preference, and act upon that instead of saying: "Nice, but we cannot do it."
>
> —Walter Flores
> Executive Director
> Center for the Study of Equity and Governance in Health Systems
> Guatemala

Those power shifts and the intent behind them must be explicit, added Bellagio participant Mao Amis, founder and executive director of the African Centre for a Green Economy. "Because of apartheid in South Africa, when they tried to do the transformation they grouped together women and people of color as disadvantaged," Amis said. "And what ended up happening is . . . white people remain in positions of power where we should actually have transformed the entire thing. In universities in South Africa, we have access of black people into the universities, but what is the quality of participation? It should be comfortable for you to come into a room like this and speak with your very strange accent without necessarily trying to fit in, as opposed to believing that you must align yourself so people can understand you."

Defining and Embracing Well-Being at the Grassroots Level

A thread running throughout the Bellagio meeting was the critical importance that what well-being means must be articulated at the grassroots level, rather than imposed by experts or governments. People in communities already have the answers to what well-being means to them. It is embedded in the wisdom traditions and the lived experiences, aspirations, hopes, and values of people all over the world. Instead of assuming that leaders will bring the well-being framework to communities, leaders should instead look at what's happening and build on what communities are already doing.

"The idea of well-being hasn't just been thought up by folks around this table," said Mallika Dutt, founder and director of the global initiative Inter-Connected, and a Bellagio participant. "It actually comes from a deep organizing among constituencies around the world. What is really important for us to remember as we move forward in this dialogue is how we continue to make sure we don't hijack or transform that conversation into our own ways of operating in the world where we make it an elite conversation."

Additionally, a benefit of engaging communities, people, and organizations as true partners in the work of defining well-being is that this engagement is a starting point for fostering grassroots demand for the implementation of a shared well-being framework. That is, a place to start movement building is to start really listening.

Participants made it clear that when they spoke about grass roots, they were thinking about constituencies across socioeconomic, geographic, demographic, and public and private sectors and fields. They envisioned engaging communities in all of their diversity and deeply thinking about fostering a dynamic process where those perspectives, experiences, and contexts are informing the well-being framework, strategies, metrics—that is, the entire approach.

At the same time, it is critical to practice radical inclusion and ensure that people from communities that are often—and have historically been—excluded from meaningful input and decision-making are engaged and contribute to an understanding of what well-being means. In addition to Indigenous communities and racial or ethnic groups, this may include those who are living in poverty, experiencing homelessness, incarcerated, struggling with substance abuse, and others.

Looking to Indigenous Cultures for Deeper Understanding of Well-Being

Many of the current notions of well-being have deep roots within Indigenous cultures, norms, and knowledge, including social cohesion and connection, intergenerational perspective, and expanding from a singular focus on the human condition to a larger connection with the environment and earth. Romlie Mokak, CEO of the Lowitja Institute in Australia, noted at Bellagio that among Indigenous peoples the health of the individual and families and the health of the earth are connected; if the health of the earth is not good, people's well-being cannot be good.

But too often, the world's 370 million Indigenous people, who live in more than 70 countries, are ignored, invisible, or reduced to stereotypes or antiquated stories rather than being seen as contemporary people with agency and ideas. Their story is told through a deficit frame of challenges and problems rather than through the lens of strength, resilience, and leadership. That is an issue for a number of reasons, among them that it will be difficult to advance a well-being framework when so many people's voice and contribution are made invisible, and when a city or country's definition of well-being—which becomes the root of measurement and action—lacks the perspective, priorities, and values of entire groups of people.

Listening by First Asking the Right Questions

To learn more about how people define well-being, it may be necessary to start by calling it something else. Well-being is not a phrase that many people use just yet—at least in the holistic way discussed at Bellagio. But the point is to get a deep understanding of what people and communities want, what will give them satisfaction in life, no matter what words they use to describe it.

One way to do this is by observing what people prioritize and take action to protect. For example, Flores noted that some grassroots groups are opposing mining in their countries, concerned that it is polluting the drinking water and the rivers that they use to grow their crops. Well-being for them is about clean drinking water and the ability to continue farming; even though mining may offer economic benefits, it is not the priority. This insight, gained by looking at actions people are taking at the community level, underscores the fact that material wealth and consumption is not seen as the path to progress for many people.

Asking people directly what well-being means for their lives and in their community will yield a much deeper and more practical understanding than simply relying on observations or objective assessments of well-being.

Anita Rajan, CEO of Tata STRIVE, noted at the Bellagio gathering that in India when she and her colleagues meet with young people and ask about their aspirations, a common theme is that money matters to them, something that was echoed by several others in attendance who see that value expressed in their countries as well. If research and wisdom show that wealth, at least alone, is not the best route to success and happiness, she asked, how do those promoting well-being respond?

Liz Zeidler, chief executive of Happy City in the United Kingdom, said that having enough money for life's basic needs is an incredibly important part of well-being. But it is not the end goal. She suggested finding the right question that gets people to tap into something a bit deeper. Ask a young person what they want, and the answer may be a new iPad because they are constantly told that acquisition of material goods is the answer to prosperity and happiness. But asking people what brings them *lasting* well-being and happiness can help get them to think about and share more profound answers.

"Just adding that word 'lasting' is a bit of a push," said Zeidler. "You're not telling them the answer but it's a push. I think it massively matters what questions we ask."

She also suggested asking people what their own family or religious traditions tell them because there are some universal elements that will draw out wisdom.

Bellagio participant Katherine Trebeck, knowledge and policy lead for the global Wellbeing Economy Alliance, said that she and fellow participant Sir Harry Burns, professor of global public health at the University of Strathclyde and Scotland's former chief medical officer, worked on a project with Oxfam in Scotland that was built around deliberative conversations with some of the most underserved communities that asked what mattered to them. To their surprise, the project delivered far more than its modest budget might have allowed, by challenging the politics around what progress looks like and the role of the government in making that a reality.

"There's an instrumental role [for public deliberation] in terms of getting political traction, if we take the time to include communities and put people's voices at the forefront," Trebeck said. "It's not just being vital in and of itself; it's also very hard for politicians to not take notice of something when you say, 'This is what a huge number of the population really wants.'"

Burns added that the Nordic School of Public Health talks a lot about salutogenesis, a medical approach focusing on factors that support human health and well-being, rather than on factors that cause disease. The salutogenic drivers are people having a sense of control over their lives and a sense of purpose. But rather than countries and cities using concepts like this to define what they should do for people to enhance their well-being, the most important thing they need to do is to ask people and communities to define their own needs for increasing their well-being. He drove home the simple but critical point, "Ask people, 'What do you need?'"

The answers they give, he said, are often simple, but that does not mean they are simplistic. Burns said if you ask someone who is homeless what they need, they are likely to tell you a new pair of glasses, a hearing aid, or something else seemingly very simple. But the system is not set up to respond to those requests. Burns said that in London, there was a homelessness project that set up bank accounts of £3,000 for each homeless person that they were serving. At the end of the year, the average spend from each account was £780. "When you ask people, 'What do you need?' you will be surprised by how modest their requests are," Burns said.

A New Model of Leadership and Decision-Making

Listening deeply and asking good questions are crucial first steps. But too often people and communities have been asked for their input only to have it ignored when it conflicts with the goals of those in power. A vital part of the process of creating a culture of well-being is taking on the hard and important work of fostering a new model of leadership and decision-making. In that model, people and organizations are not chosen simply to represent a constituency, but they have, and exercise, real power.

Flores said that the most important task in this work is to build a constituency that will demand and put pressure on the authorities to move forward a well-being framework. But that must be done by first recognizing the real dynamics at play and then taking deliberate steps to shake up those dynamics so that those who have had less power will have real decision-making impact. He noted that an issue with the well-being framework is that it is power blind. For Flores, that is a major weakness because a true breakthrough in advancing a well-being movement will require alliances of different constituencies and social mobilization strategies that will challenge power relations. But for those alliances to take hold, participants must grapple with issues of power, including power differentials in those alliances and how to shift them—and ultimately to make real shifts in power.

"The well-being agenda framework concept, as unifying and as inclusive as it might be conceptually, at its heart is a radical departure from the current status quo," said Dutt. "And as we all know, status quo doesn't just shift quickly and easily because people think that it should. We're not trying to articulate well-being as some sort of a kumbaya moment where we all come together and hold hands and dance around the fire, but really to understand that what we are talking about is a radical shift in what is, and to hold ourselves accountable to that radical shift. [We need to] make sure that we do not hide or run away from the very deep [power] relationship questions as we move forward the well-being agenda."

Building engagement, ownership, and trust

A departure of this magnitude takes time, and a commitment to stay the course. Systems that value efficiency, particularly government systems, are set up for control, not listening to and acting on people's perspectives and needs, so true engagement is often seen as a lot of extra work. But a number of examples exist where organizations have undertaken extensive public engagement and—importantly—taken that engagement on board in their well-being planning processes.

Happy City, a U.K. charity that seeks to refocus measures and actions on well-being and what matters most, spent two to three years in the heart of communities including schools, prisons, shopping centers, businesses, and community halls to learn from people what mattered to them, and what well-being looked like in practice. Happy City took this information and fed it into its Thriving Places Index. Leaders also consulted experts and people working on the front line, such as in NGOs, to test and get feedback on each step they took. Importantly, a guiding principle for the charity's work is, does it have meaning for people living at the margins of society as well as top local policymakers.

A key reframe that emerged in the discussion of real grassroots engagement at Bellagio was addressing head-on and completely shifting the perspective of those in power toward grassroots activists. Often policymakers, organizational leaders, and others with influence can see those who bring a different point of view, who demand changes in process, who question existing definitions, and who see different solutions as slowing down the process or being part of the problem that must be solved. Participants at Bellagio suggested the need to, instead, see them as problem solvers who can make a real difference rather than dismissing them. Doing so not only taps into their wisdom and identity, but also helps flip the script. They are not the cause of problems—they hold the solutions. This is particularly important for young people, especially adolescents, who can be easily ignored.

Engaging Youth as Leaders in the Well-Being Movement

A key thread throughout the meeting was the need to more deliberately engage young people in the well-being movement. This approach focuses on the future and long-term change, making it inherently a multi-generational effort, and young people will both lead new solutions and bear the consequences of decisions made today. Young people can bring fresh eyes, perspectives, and energy to well-being initiatives, including doing what they do best: critiquing and changing the status quo. Youth leadership around the world on climate change provides a strong example of the power of this approach.

Participants shared stories from Singapore, Nova Scotia, Bhutan, Australia, and the United Arab Emirates about efforts to identify the pathway for millennials to understand and take leadership roles in well-being-focused decision-making. In Australia, Mokak explained, the Lowitja Institute has been instrumental in supporting a new generation of Aboriginal and Torres Strait Islander health researchers who bring early-career perspectives to research, policy, and services. And the Australian Indigenous Doctors' Association, which he led for nearly a decade, is training a new generation of young Indigenous doctors who could lead the way to more a culturally relevant and trusted health system, addressing the systemic racism that contributes to severe and persistent disparities. "Our young people felt a huge amount of pressure in being Indigenous in a completely different cultural context [in medical school]," Mokak says. "In many cases, people were told to leave their Indigenous culture at the door because it was now a culture of medicine that they needed to be integrated into." The Australian Indigenous Doctors' Association supports medical students in building strength and resilience and being "almost activists in their approach," Mokak said, to changing the status quo. Further, Indigenous leaders in Australia are drawing on traditional practices and ceremonies in growing their leaders of the future. They are providing youth with mentoring and support, in both Indigenous cultural ways and professional practice, to equip them to cope with the many leadership demands early in their careers.

> *If we really want to change, then we've got to start investing in the new gener-*
> *ation, and that new generation builds into new leadership.*
> *—Nancy Wildfeir-Field*
> *President*
> *GBCHealth*
> *United States and Africa*

In Bhutan, the GNH Centre is working with students and young people to help them articulate and understand Gross National Happiness (GNH) for themselves so that they view it not as something that's to be kept in a museum but as a concept they can bring into their own lives and community. Bellagio participant Julia Kim, program director of the GNH Centre Bhutan, shared the example of the Loden Foundation, which is encouraging a growing entrepreneurial community to create small businesses inspired by GNH values. In supporting and coaching these youth, they make reference to the notion of a "bodhisattva entrepreneur," evoking the image of a Buddhist hero who has the motivation of serving society, and starts a business as a means to that end.

Participants also spoke about engaging universities as leaders in the well-being movement. Because their mission is educating young people and preparing them for the world, higher education leaders hold a unique position of influence in moving a well-being framework forward. In Singapore, one of the initiatives to enhance well-being is the Healthy Campus Initiative, which will be launched at two major universities there. A deep-seated value in Singapore, like other places, is to equate wealth with success. The Healthy Campus Initiative aims to shift this, creating a cohort of university graduates by 2025 who operate with a different mindset.

"These are graduates who [will] value health just as much as wealth," said Bellagio participant Kee-Seng Chia, founding dean of the National University of Singapore's School of Public Health. "They will continue to be lifelong health investors, creating social movement for healthy living, and they will be healthier when they leave the campus than when they first came in."

A well-being frame may also open opportunities for education systems to address issues that have been uncomfortable or they have not understood how to address. Those include sexual violence, equity, and racism.

Shifting Power

Participants said that they and other advocates can put all the new dials on the dashboard, backed up by the most rigorous evidence, but if they do not address power and inequities in who has decision-making authority, the well-being framework will sputter and never truly take off. Several participants noted that the response to including Indigenous and other marginalized populations is often to create representation, which can feel like tokenism. When someone "representing" a community has one vote in a body of 60, that is not real power.

Flores pointed out that different groups have varying degrees of power, and understanding that landscape will inform the best strategies to influence changes. For example, in the case of Indigenous populations, the main sources of power are sovereign territories, which can be used for negotiations when land is targeted for a pipeline or water rights. Migrants who come to the United States from Latin America have power because their labor is needed; minority populations in Eastern Europe, such as the Roma population, on the other hand, do not have the same potential sway because they are not seen as necessary to the economy. When Indigenous knowledge is valued, as it can and should be in the well-being movement, that knowledge creates power.

Another important aspect of shifting power is to help people see their own leadership capacity in ways that they might not have before—and to help leaders in a colonized or dominant system recognize that leadership does not have to look the same in every context. In a world where power is often equated with people in charge of governments and corporations, the notion of power must be recast.

"From my experience, what I try to instill in people who I'm cultivating as leaders is the idea that power is definitely not titular power and it's not hierarchical power," said Bellagio participant Claire Nelson, lead futurist of the Futures Forum in the United States and the Caribbean. "And my experience as a change-maker is that I never had either of those. What I had was what I call my 'passion power' and a sense of moral imperative if you will. And if this issue is a moral imperative for human survival, I think with enough people—it doesn't have to be everybody—enough people can move the agenda."

Power shifts must happen in all spaces where power is at play: government, business, finance, academia, the nonprofit sector, and all other aspects of society. Of the many ways people and organizations can be mobilized for change, shareholder actions were identified as one to consider. As an example, efforts to shift use of plastics were led by the communities facing the most environmental degradation and health impacts; demands to diversify corporate boards are being driven by advocates and customers. Changes in business practices can also shift power: Consider fair-trade coffee certification to provide greater income and better conditions for coffee workers. Legal actions are another pathway; for example, tribes with sovereignty can sue on issues around natural resources (e.g., the Keystone Pipeline) or use treaty rights with veto power on issues ranging from protecting fisheries to water rights. Media and social media can be employed to bring attention *and* change, as tribes did with Standing Rock, and as activists—and their followers—did with Black Lives Matter, #MeToo, and other movements.

The bottom line is that simply making changes within existing decision-making structures is not enough to create needed shifts in power to address injustice and advance broadly shared well-being. It is crucial to establish new decision-making rights and systems that provide representation with power.

Building Pressure From the Grassroots for Decision-Makers to Take New Actions

For the well-being framework to become rooted in the ways government, business, education, the nonprofit sector, and others approach their work, it is incumbent to engage people who can have influence from a number of different positions and perspectives. Those include people within the system holding formalized positions of power, people who have informal positions as influencers, and those advocating from outside of a system who can demand change.

A huge task—and the most important one going forward—is to build diverse constituencies who will demand advances in an equitable well-being framework.

Conclusion

Effective engagement of diverse constituencies, deep listening to the grass roots, and real shifts in power will influence the success of all other work discussed in this volume. And while these concepts are fundamental to many social movements, participants at Bellagio recognized how intrinsically important they are to advancing well-being. This work will define well-being and inform measurement, surface ideas to lift up and spread across sectors, and influence the narrative by shaping the narrative itself as well as building public will.

If these important steps are not taken, advocates for a well-being framework run the real risk of repeating the old top-down solutions that not only do not speak to the deepest needs of grassroots communities, but also lack the wisdom, depth, and nuance that they would have if this engagement had taken place. Conversely, deeply engaging with and valuing the grassroots community and addressing power dynamics head-on holds the real promise of moving the well-being framework forward in ways that are informed by both academic research and the wisdom of lived experience, and with inclusive decision-making that can ensure changes truly take hold.

SECTION V

BREAKING DOWN SILOS AND ENCOURAGING INNOVATION

Advancing well-being requires leadership, innovation, and action in every sector. It has relevance to and can benefit from the work of many movements and opens spaces for cross-sector collaboration. It creates opportunities—even a mandate—to rethink the way fields' departments are structured, bringing them from isolation to integration. After all, the challenges a well-being approach seeks to address don't fit neatly in one box; neither, then, can the solutions.

Governments are forming new cross-agency positions and initiatives to lead well-being efforts, or, as Bellagio participant and deputy secretary and chief economic adviser of the New Zealand Treasury, Tim Ng, discusses in chapter 9, structuring entire government budgets and planning processes around the well-being construct. Corporations, funders, nongovernmental organizations, and others across civil society are asking different questions about how to set goals, measure outcomes, and chart a course for the future. This interplay between government and other sectors is vital; well-being-driven policy can be advanced or undermined by advocacy, market choices, and private sector practices. Or innovation driven by the private sector and NGOs can create transformative opportunities from how we grow our food to how we power our communities, but without an aligned policy environment these innovations cannot come to scale.

A well-being approach draws on broad, discipline-spanning indicators to assess and address human and societal conditions. It challenges entrenched approaches in science and research, government and policymaking, funding streams, and elsewhere. It encourages collaboration among health, economics, development, environmental protection, housing, social services, education, and many other fields. Through a well-being lens, a deeper, more dynamic framing unfolds about how people interact with systems and environments and the impact that has on their ability to flourish.

Vital opportunities exist to change incentives, systems, and structures across all sectors to create space for innovation. In government, there is opportunity to move from an activity- and field-driven structure—for example, education, health, and labor—to outcome- and impact-driven models, such as vibrant and equitable communities, individual and family well-being, and economic mobility. Many public sector examples of well-being approaches are rooted in applying measurement and policy screens to see how decisions will impact well-being. Discussion and experimentation is establishing that this is not just about changing the gauge on the dashboard or creating new justification for the same old action; it's about rebuilding programs, systems, and structures to advance well-being.

Alongside government, the private sector has significant influence ranging from information flow and the narratives advanced in pop culture, to human settlement patterns and the function of core systems, such as food, energy, and health care. The participants at Bellagio identified opportunities where the private sector could be a catalyst for advancing well-being, from accelerating the use of Environmental, Social, and Governance (ESG) considerations (particularly in embedding well-being indicators in the "S" social element), to updating industry standards and good practices to align with well-being outcomes. Discussion also explored the potential for private sector practices to benefit from a well-being approach, including rapid prototyping; systems innovation to meet demands created by increased well-being expectations; and the ongoing reach through supply chains, employees, customers, and marketing.

Philanthropy and nongovernmental organizations are a third sector whose mission-driven mandate aligns with many of the tenets of well-being, including the emphasis on equity. This sector often has more freedom to experiment than the public sector and more ability to invest in non-monetized exploration than the private sector. Bellagio participants discussed in depth the power, potential, and barriers for this sector in focusing on well-being, ranging from the need to shift funding and programs to advance well-being outcomes, to using their power as institutional investors and influencers of new action. Several case studies and many of the examples of grassroots engagement and innovation described NGOs that are, or could be, serving as trusted intermediaries and effective advocates.

There is a highly appealing value proposition here: Because well-being is more inclusive than purely economic-driven progress indicators and takes a systemic and prevention-based approach, it has the potential to create new alignment and efficiencies in all sectors.

In chapter 9, "Creating a Government Commitment to Well-Being," Ng reviews how New Zealand developed the Living Standards Framework (LSF), an economic framework that includes well-being outcomes on a population level. The LSF is influencing strategic fiscal and economic policy advice, and demonstrates a real-world example of the well-being approach in action at a national government level.

Chapter 10, "Opportunities Across Every Sector to Advance a Well-Being Framework: Discussion and Case Studies From Bellagio," shares insights about advancing well-being across sectors at local, national, and international levels. It explores other public sector examples and shares insights on key motivators, levers for impact, and potential challenges for the private, nongovernmental, and philanthropic sectors in advancing a well-being approach.

Creating a Government Commitment to Well-Being

TIM NG
Deputy Secretary and Chief Economic Adviser
*The New Zealand Treasury**

New Zealand is a developed country of five million people in the South Pacific, with a substantial Indigenous (Māori) population and bicultural governance foundations as expressed in the Treaty of Waitangi of 1840. It has a long tradition of debate on big questions about social, environmental, and economic well-being—and about the link between them. After some years of developing analytical tools and approaches to addressing these questions, the New Zealand Government in 2019 demonstrated its commitment to well-being as a public policy principle with the release of its Wellbeing Budget. Launching the Wellbeing Budget, Prime Minister Jacinda Ardern said, "When [Minister of Finance Grant Robertson] heard many an economist say that GDP wasn't enough to measure success he agreed and did something about it . . . [t]oday we further our shared ambition to ensure all New Zealanders do well, but especially our children . . . [this] Government is not satisfied with the status quo and instead is tackling our long-term challenges."[1]

This chapter discusses how the New Zealand Treasury's Living Standards Framework (LSF) has guided the Treasury's policy advice to governments in

* The author is grateful to Paul Dalziel, Arthur Grimes, Nicholas Gruen, and Fiona Ross for helpful discussions on the ideas expressed in this chapter. All errors and omissions remain the author's. The views, opinions, findings, and conclusions or recommendations expressed in this chapter are strictly those of the author. They do not necessarily reflect the views of the New Zealand Treasury or the New Zealand Government. The New Zealand Treasury and the New Zealand Government take no responsibility for any errors or omissions in, or for the correctness of, the information contained in the chapter.

New Zealand, using the Wellbeing Budget as a key example of the application of the LSF in practice. The LSF is a population-level economic framework with a multidimensional well-being outcomes focus and associated measurement, analysis, and assessment tools. It helps the government to express, analyze, and implement its well-being objectives in the form of concrete policy action. As well as government budget management, the LSF has been applied to strategic fiscal and economic policy development.[2]

The framework has informed debate about sustainable development; helped shine a light on the most pressing social, environmental, and economic concerns facing the country; and provided an analytical structure within which to consider and assess potential government responses across multiple agencies. Priority policy areas for funding and other interventions that were identified through this process and addressed in the Wellbeing Budget included mental health, family and sexual violence, and sustainable land use.

In this chapter, we discuss some of the learnings, opportunities, and challenges to date in the development and use of the LSF, and some thoughts on future directions. The chapter begins with an overview of the creation and use of the LSF, then elaborates in three sections. The next section describes the conceptual essentials of the LSF, including a diagram of its core components and indicators and the approach to using it to support policy. Section 2 looks at the experience of applying LSF tools to various stages of the policy process, including examples of cross-agency collaboration and the resulting policy packages informed by the LSF. Finally, section 3 discusses the work still needed over the coming years to embed well-being principles firmly at the core of government policy and action in New Zealand.

Overview of This Chapter

The LSF was formally introduced in 2011, and can be understood as a waypoint in a larger process of increasing focus in New Zealand, as well as other developed countries, on broadening economic, fiscal, and regulatory analysis to recognize more explicitly the ultimate well-being objectives of public policy. The early documentation articulated the Treasury's conception of the connection between economic performance, government intervention, and living standards, or well-being.[3] The LSF at its inception was, and still is, influenced by a number of strands of thinking.

First, its philosophical foundations derive from the "capabilities" approach substantially developed by Amartya Sen and Martha Nussbaum, which has the concept of freedom at its heart. In this worldview, freedom to achieve well-being is a matter of what people are able to do and to be, and thus the kind of life they are effectively able to lead.[3,4]

Second, the work draws on literature reframing or reconfirming economic policy as being ultimately about the enduring high-level, multidimensional well-being outcomes representing human flourishing.[5,6]

Third, the work responds to the perceived inadequacies of traditional, compartmentalized policy approaches to confront complex contemporary challenges, such as rapid technological change, social disconnection and disparities, environmental degradation, and climate change.[7,8]

Finally, given the objective of practical application, the day-to-day demands of policy agencies and applied knowledge of international policy institutions, such as the Organisation for Economic Co-operation and Development (OECD), have been relevant.[2]

The LSF maintains a key role for "traditional" economic policy approaches that seek to strengthen both the capabilities of people to participate in formal labor markets, and the productivity gains resulting from market processes, recognizing that these are fundamental means of lifting real incomes and life opportunities. Both of these outcomes are critical foundations of well-being: Higher incomes enable households and communities to pursue well-being on their own terms; and well-crafted policies promoting well-functioning labor and goods markets have driven the strong association between incomes and well-being evident across the ages.[9] Such policies will always be an important core of what governments do.

Building on that base, the LSF sharpens the focus in policy development on causally linking well-being outcomes to potential intervention options. The explicit well-being starting point recognizes more systematically and coherently that strong economic performance is only a means (albeit a very important means) to the end of higher well-being. It confronts the notion that for some policy challenges and interventions, sharp tradeoffs and interdependencies across different well-being dimensions can be highly salient at the population, community, household, and individual levels. This is especially relevant when human activities in production, labor, and consumption markets encroach on the limits of environmental and social acceptability. Such cases raise choices, on which the LSF can shed analytical light, about how to fix or supplement the markets (possibly with new markets) and how to compensate administratively for adverse effects of market activities.

The development and application of the LSF is consistent with calls from international organizations, such as the OECD[10] and the World Bank,[11] for governments to enrich their policies toward principles of sustainability and intergenerational well-being. A number of OECD governments are now using broad well-being concepts in their policy narratives, and government-curated "dashboards" of well-being measures are common. Experience in a range of jurisdictions, such as France, Germany, Italy, and Sweden, is also now emerging with the use of the measures in policy processes.[10,12,13] New Zealand is a participant in the now-regular international discussions on the well-being agenda, seeking to exchange perspectives, insights, and successful practices.

Building on the inception of the LSF some years earlier, the incoming New Zealand government in 2017 expressed an intention to develop and use broader "measures of success" that went beyond traditional economic indicators, and to embed principles of well-being throughout its policy program. Its intended reforms included changes to government and official reporting requirements about well-being, governance arrangements for the public sector, and the processes by which government agencies develop policy advice and deliver government services (all underway at the time of writing). As a first major step in this program, the government explicitly drew on the LSF to support the development of the 2019 "Wellbeing Budget,"[14] an innovation that received global media attention.[15,16] This application by the incoming government drove a substantial shift up in the intensity of work on the LSF.

Using in actual policy practice a framework such as the LSF—which is still in development, and where the body of knowledge is incomplete in many respects—is challenging. Many uncharted waters remain. The further development of the LSF will be emergent and adaptive, and will need to draw on experience and ideas from a wide range of sources. In particular, while approaches to measuring population-level well-being appear essentially sufficient to support current policy application, processes for using the indicators to develop, prioritize, and evaluate new policy initiatives specifically in terms of well-being are just beginning, and are considerably less mature.

Conceptual Essentials of the LSF

Three roles for "progress" indicators

The use of the broad capability-based framing partly reflects the Treasury's role, as part of the professional public service, in providing advice to successive governments about economic and fiscal performance. The LSF constructively supports two of the three roles for progress indicators defined in Rondinella (2014):[17] first, an *instrumental* role to support better policy decisions through the analytical policy advice process, and second, a *conceptual* or discursive role to define terms in particular narratives or framings of policy problems. The framework plays these two roles by providing an evidence-based common language for analysts.

Rondinella's third role is a *political* role about the ways in which governments build a sense of legitimacy and mandate to pursue their policy programs. Being clear about the meaning of well-being, both conceptually and empirically, enables governments to hold themselves to account for the outcomes they are trying to achieve, and to engage others in debate about different public policy choices. In the process, governments must apply, as elected representatives, essentially political value judgments, preferences, and priorities across a range of well-being domains. The Treasury's need to keep its policy advice politically neutral means being careful that the LSF's choice of indicators and conceptual framing can accommodate the various values and priorities of both current and future New Zealand governments. These priorities frame the policies on which the Treasury can expect to be called to advise. The framework needs to support advice in the nexus between economic and fiscal performance and a wide range of other concerns, including social and environmental issues and matters of rights and freedoms. In order for the framework to be useful and to endure, it needs to avoid its choices of domains and concepts inadvertently constraining or intruding on political actors' preferred policy narratives, while at the same time remaining anchored in evidence.

An accommodative approach

An accommodative, capability-based view of what enables individuals, households, and communities to flourish also helps to draw in different perspectives, traditions, and cultures to think about and evaluate different approaches to promoting well-being. The approach can support older Western approaches to the economics of human welfare that emerged in the latter stages of the Enlightenment, such as the "utilitarian" approach associated with Jeremy Bentham and J. S. Mill, in which the proper objective of government is seen to be the promotion of "the greatest good for the greatest number."[18] But the LSF has also supported the Treasury's engagement with New Zealand communities whose value systems have elements or structures that are in some respects distinct from those derived from Western traditions. The development of the LSF has consequently been informed by a range of consultations with ethnic community groups directly, as well as with expert scholars. For example, engagement with Māori (Indigenous New Zealand) people in the context of policy development has helped clarify the elements of the Māori worldview most relevant and connected to well-being.[19,20] Similar, but not identical, themes emerged from discussions with Pacific[21] and Asian[22] people on their perspectives. Understanding the role of culture, cultural expression, and cultural artifacts as important sources of well-being, irrespective of cultural origins, is also germane to the development of the framework.[23]

In practice, for the narrow purposes of choosing well-being domains and indicators at the aggregate level, theoretical underpinnings appear not to matter too much.[24] The domains and indicators of well-being in a range of frameworks reviewed by King et al. (2018)[25] covered a similar range of social, economic, and environmental conditions. They are also the kinds of factors that members of the New Zealand public nominated when the Treasury engaged in a focus-group exercise about the "things that matter" during an early application of the LSF.[26]

However, at the level of *distribution* of well-being within the aggregates, the underpinnings can make a difference to the focus of inquiry. For example, the capabilities-based view sharpens the focus on individuals, households, or communities as the relevant actors, or their experiences as the relevant units of analysis, whereas a simple utilitarian view might emphasize national aggregates and per capita averages. A Māori or Pacific worldview would place strong emphasis on the well-being of the wider family and tribal group as the unit of analysis, and on the well-being of the environment as inseparable from the well-being of humanity.

Further, the emphasis on what people are able to do and to be supports analysis of the relational or procedural aspects of well-being, which are also important in New Zealand. Its founding governance document, the Treaty of Waitangi between the British Crown and Indigenous Māori iwi (tribes),* defines relations between the two parties. The meaning of the rights and obligations embodied in the Treaty and subsequently given expression in civic and political life animates much contemporary debate about culture and well-being in New Zealand. At the level of individual behavior and what makes for a good life, Māori perspectives on well-being tend to emphasize such behavioral aspects of life as knowing one's ancestry, exercising rights to knowledge, and expressing culture through acts such as recounting traditional narratives. Te Rito (2006)[27] provides an extensive discussion of indigeneity and well-being in the New Zealand context, while the broader issues of culture and well-being are discussed in Dalziel, Saunders, and Savage (2019).[23]

The LSF domains and structure in summary

Notwithstanding the different theoretical and cultural perspectives that the LSF at least aspires to accommodate, the design of the specific well-being taxonomy

---

* In Aotearoa New Zealand usage, the Māori language term "iwi" (Māori pronunciation: [ˈiwi]) means extended kinship group, tribe, nation, people, nationality, race. It is often translated as "tribe" or "a confederation of tribes" and typically refers to a large group of people descended from a common ancestor and associated with a distinct territory. The word is both singular and plural in Māori.

in the 2019 version of the LSF has been influenced most directly by the OECD's Better Life Initiative, reflecting the Initiative's focus on improving the evidence base to support policy—a more or less identical objective to the Treasury's in developing the LSF. The Treasury has adapted and augmented the 11 fundamental current well-being domains in the *How's Life?* approach within the Initiative to suit New Zealand's circumstances, and added a 12th domain to cover the relevance of cultural identity to well-being in New Zealand. The way in which society's resources support the well-being of future generations is recognized by "four capitals" (financial/physical, human, social, and natural). These capitals can be interpreted as stocks of productive resources that are used by human actors to produce flows of well-being, analogously to the way in which built capital (factories, buildings, infrastructure, etc.) is used to produce market income in a traditional economic framework. The distribution of well-being across the population, different population subgroups and regions; risks to well-being and the resilience of the capitals to adverse shocks; and the dynamism of the economic system to respond to threats and opportunities all have a place in the framework. See **Figure 1**.

Figure 1. The New Zealand Treasury's Living Standards Framework

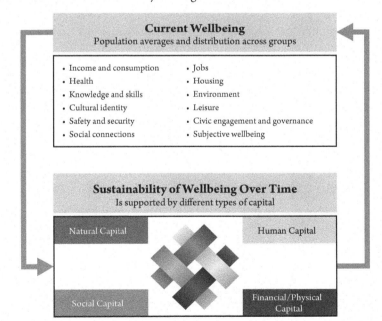

In this figure, *natural capital* refers to all aspects of the natural environment that support life and human activity, including land, soil, water, plants and animals, minerals, and energy resources. *Human capital* refers to the capabilities and

capacities of people to engage in work, study, recreation, and social activities, including skills, knowledge, and physical and mental health. *Social capital* refers to the norms, rules, and institutions that influence the way in which people live and work together and experience a sense of belonging, including trust, reciprocity, the rule of law, cultural and community identity, traditions and customs, and common values and interests. *Financial and physical capital* refers to financial and human-made physical assets, usually closely associated with supporting material living conditions, including factories, equipment, houses, roads, buildings, hospitals, and financial securities.

The close connection between the LSF and the OECD framework enables comparison of New Zealand's experience with a well-being agenda against those of other developed countries. It also helps analysts connect to the OECD's considerable body of well-being research and analysis of the impacts of well-being and other policy, and vice versa. For example, in 2019, the OECD's regular review of New Zealand, the *Country Survey*, featured an extensive assessment of both well-being itself in New Zealand, and the state of play in the use of the LSF.[28]

The examination of the framework in an internationally high-profile policy assessment process, such as the *Country Survey*, helps embed it within government policy processes and sharpen thinking about how evidence for a well-being approach can be used best to guide policy. Recognizing that applying a well-being framework to policy development remains at an early stage in New Zealand, the 2019 *Country Survey* noted that the data and evidence base require further development, and that civil service implementation capacity needs strengthening. The New Zealand authorities intend to continue to work closely with the OECD on these issues, which should help both parties and strengthen the body of evidence for other countries and organizations to draw on.

The Application of the LSF in New Zealand Government Processes

2017 marks a shift in the prominence of the LSF as a policy development tool

Until the formation of the new Labour-led Government in 2017, the LSF was mainly an internally-focused capability development work program in the Treasury. It was focused on upskilling its analysts to tackle contemporary multidimensional and complex policy issues. Some associated assessment tools, guidance, and heuristics to help analysts think through different aspects of policy assessment were in use and development to support parts of the previous government's program. These included extensive guidance on the use of cost-benefit analysis to address non-monetary impacts, and the related "Cost Benefit Analysis eXtra" (CBAx) modeling tool. CBAx enables quantitative (including monetized) assessment of dynamic and non-monetary costs and benefits of investment proposals.[29] Although various LSF-related materials and applications were published during that period, the profile of the LSF beyond the Treasury and a small number of interested practitioners and observers in Wellington was modest.

The government of the time also did not use the LSF explicitly as an organizing principle in its policy development processes, which limited other government agencies' interest in it. Notwithstanding that, some of the core ideas common to both the LSF and the government's "Social Investment" social policy program were clearly present in the government's articulation of what it was trying to achieve (see e.g., previous minister of finance, Bill English [2016]).[30] These included the importance of considering life course and intergenerational impacts of policy and government service interventions across multiple dimensions, and the importance of cross-agency coordination to deliver effective results in complex social circumstances.

After the 2017 general election, the prominence of the LSF in guiding policy and policy processes increased significantly as the incoming Labour-led Coalition Government announced plans to use it as a core analytical tool in its policy agenda.[31] The earlier work enabled the Treasury to respond quickly to this demand, and the Government to refer to some actual practice, tools, and thinking that already existed within the Treasury. The minister of finance recognized, though, that further development work was needed to support what the government wanted to do with the framework (see his remarks at the time, cited below).

The government's reference to wider well-being thinking of the sort described in the introduction to this chapter was evident in the way in which the public narrative on well-being unfolded in the political process. Prior to the election, the Labour Party had campaigned with a policy narrative that emphasized traditionally-conceived economic and fiscal performance as necessary, but not sufficient, for success in terms of overall well-being. In the words of the Labour Party leader and later prime minister, Jacinda Ardern, in the context of the Labour party's fiscal policy agenda, "building a strong economy is not enough to declare success," while the finance spokesperson (later minister of finance) Grant Robertson connected success explicitly to the concept of well-being, stating the Party's intention to "ensure that the budgets we produce are not just narrow fiscal documents. We will measure our success in how we improve the well-being of all New Zealanders, how we are reducing child poverty and improving sustainability. We will always remember that our fiscal plan is merely the means to the end of supporting New Zealanders to have lives of dignity, security, and hope."[32]

Subsequent to the formation of the new government, the minister of finance expressed how he intended to use the LSF at that stage of its development as follows:[33]

> At the moment the LSF is transitioning from the theoretical to the practical. As the LSF is refined into a robust tool, it will help us answer questions about:
>
> - The health of the four capitals—natural, human, social, and physical/ financial—and whether or not they are growing and likely to be sustained.
> - Social and demographic inequalities in well-being, how the flow of current benefits affects long-term outcomes.
> - How resource allocation decisions affect capital to improve current or long-term well-being.

Accelerated development work

To meet the government's ambitions, the Treasury accelerated its work on developing the framework and associated tools and processes. As noted, some versions of the tools (particularly those used for the development and assessment of certain budget initiatives and investment proposals, and for strategic economic policy development work by the Treasury) had already been used earlier under the previous government. However, what was needed was a more cohesive and thorough articulation of the different elements of the framework and how they fit together, as well as modification of the tools themselves and how they were to be used in the policy process. This articulation and design work was needed both to support practical application much more systematically in a major government policy process (the budget), and to provide depth to the government's policy narrative.

Some practical consequences of the design work on the budget process were as follows. First, there was a stronger emphasis on cross-minister and cross-government agency engagement and deliberation as a way of focusing energy on the development of initiative packages that would best target the government's budget priorities taken as a collective. Second, the budget development process and interaction between ministers, the Treasury, and other government agencies were reorganized to bring forward by some months the step of communicating the priorities to agencies. This helped to frame and target their work on developing initiatives with more time for the necessary deliberation over the interpretation of the evidence and design of packages. Finally, as part of strengthening the emphasis on evidence, the process made more extensive use of scientific experts within agencies early in the process to provide input on the specification of priorities.

As well as this work focused on the reorganization of government policy processes around the well-being theme, the Treasury also stepped up its public communications and engagement on the LSF. It produced a number of discussion and consultation papers elaborating on the elements of the LSF, and developed a measurement dashboard for use in the policy process, which was subsequently released to the public at the end of 2018. The process of consultation attracted a wide range of commentary, mostly supportive and constructive, though it also revealed the very broad conceptions of well-being and influences on it held by different parts of the community.[2]

Improved and new tools

The Dashboard adds living standards reporting to support agenda-setting and the enrichment of existing macroeconomic and fiscal reporting documents produced by the Treasury such as the Budget Economic and Fiscal Update (BEFU) and Financial Statements of the Government. The choice of indicators and data in the Dashboard, which was informed by public and expert consultations through 2018 on a proposal paper,[24] is intended to support advice and deliberation on each of the areas of the LSF. Current social, economic, and environmental well-being conditions can be analyzed in terms of whether outcomes are worse or better than in comparator countries, whether the outcomes are trending better or worse, the states of the capitals, and so on.

For all parts of the policy process, the LSF is intended to promote the use of common measures and language, and an integrated causal view of how well-being evolves over time and is influenced by government action. The LSF augments and enriches existing Treasury tools for economic and fiscal policy analysis and development. "Traditional" finance ministry concerns for value for money, economic performance and productivity, and fiscal prudence and macroeconomic stability remain, of course. There is nothing particularly new about the ideas that well-being does not derive from monetary considerations alone, and that there are methodological limits to how useful "monetization" strategies can be as analytical tools for comparing quite different outcome alternatives. But the value added by the LSF is to bring together more consistently the range of relevant knowledge and analytical tools, and to contribute to policy coherence. As the OECD[34] puts it, policy coherence is a state in which "the economic, social, environmental, and governance dimensions of sustainable development [are integrated] at all stages of policy making . . . [aims include to] (1) foster synergies and address trade-offs across policy areas; (2) reconcile domestic policy objectives with internationally agreed objectives; and (3) address the transboundary and long-term impacts of policies."

To provide more detail on how the LSF has been used thus far in the policy process, the following provides some examples of its application in: (1) diagnosis and agenda setting; (2) proposal generation, assessment, and resource allocation; and (3) monitoring and evaluation.

Diagnosis and agenda setting

Since the introduction of the LSF in the early 2010s, the Treasury has sought to use the LSF explicitly in strategic economic performance assessments, which play a role in helping to frame longer-term thinking and agenda-setting by the government. Its briefing to the incoming minister of finance in 2014 drew on the themes of prosperity, sustainability, and inclusion to organize analysis of the medium-term opportunities and challenges to economic performance.[35] Its 2014 statement on the government's long-term fiscal position supplemented 40-year fiscal projections with a discussion of challenges for future living standards in New Zealand in terms of the four capitals, and illustrated the nexus between fiscal and social outcomes with quantitative modeling.[36] And its 2018 investment statement reported on the state and management of the government balance sheet and public assets, with discussion of the connection to well-being, the four capitals, and a particular focus on natural capital.[37]

Other New Zealand government agencies also maintain domain-, population-, or sector-specific reporting under their own outcomes frameworks, which supplement the LSF as a "macro level" view. Examples include the Whanau Ora Outcomes Framework for Māori,[38] the Government Policy Statement on Land Transport,[39] the New Zealand Environmental Reporting Framework (Ministry for the Environment and StatsNZ), and the Social Report (Ministry of Social Development). These disaggregated measurement frameworks in some cases define the relevant strategic outcomes sought, and feed into the agenda-setting process alongside LSF-based information.

The Wellbeing Budget agenda-setting process brought together the LSF dashboard indicator information, expert evidence, and government agency input to support collaborative discussions among ministers about the budget priorities. In doing so, it was one of the key government processes expressing the themes of more comprehensive well-being measurement and the transformation of public administration to confront complex policy challenges.[14,40]

The five budget priorities were set out in the *Budget Policy Statement*,[33] a strategic document that the government is required to publish several months ahead of the budget itself, and incorporated into the Treasury's guidance issued to agencies defining the process and parameters for initiative development and assessment.[41] The guidance was sent out about eight months before the budget, and supported and gave focus to the government's desire for a more collaborative and coherent development of packages of initiatives by ministers, through a common evidence base and language.[42]

The priorities are shown in **Box 1**.[42] The government's assessment of well-being circumstances and prospects using the LSF and other evidence was documented in a new chapter in the budget document, the "Wellbeing Outlook," alongside the macroeconomic and fiscal analysis that typically features in budget documentation.

Box 1. 2019 Wellbeing Budget Priorities

Taking Mental Health Seriously—Supporting mental well-being for all New Zealanders, with a special focus on under-24-year-olds.
Improving Child Well-Being—Reducing child poverty and improving child well-being, including addressing family violence.
Supporting Māori and Pasifika Aspirations—Lifting Māori and Pacific incomes, skills, and opportunities.
Building a Productive Nation—Supporting a thriving nation in the digital age through innovation [and] social and economic opportunities.
Transforming the Economy—Creating opportunities for productive businesses, regions, iwi, and others to transition to a sustainable and low-emissions economy.

Proposal generation, assessment, and prioritization/resource allocation

The proposal generation and assessment phase for the Wellbeing Budget 2019 also drew on LSF concepts to promote consistency and coherence in identifying where payoffs to government investment or intervention may be highest. For this phase, the minister of finance indicated his approach to using the LSF as follows:[33]

The Living Standards Framework will also have an impact on how agencies develop policy advice and deliver services. Well-being indicators should sharpen further the focus the public service has on:

- better understanding what will make a difference to well-being
- using good data and tools like a refined and revised CBAx ["Cost Benefit Analysis eXtra," the modeling tool described above] to test the likely effectiveness of policy options
- evaluating the real-life outcomes that particular services and spending are achieving—or where they are missing the mark

Lastly, the Living Standards Framework will support government agencies to work together in a cohesive way so that public policy on well-being, spending, and other government interventions are aligned to improving intergenerational well-being.

These principles are relevant to all areas of government activity (spending, investment, service delivery, regulation). To emphasize the point that well-being should not be considered to be solely about government spending, the Wellbeing Budget packages featured non-spending as well as spending initiatives. The Treasury's budget guidance required agencies to be clear about which well-being domains or capitals their initiatives were most relevant to, how the initiatives would be expected to impact positively on well-being, options analysis, the relevant evidence supporting the claimed impacts, and how the initiatives would be implemented and evaluated. The submitting agency was also required to show how it had collaborated with related agencies and ministers to develop the initiatives.

The Wellbeing Budget document set out packages of initiatives organized under each of the five priorities. These packages illustrated the well-being outcome considerations supporting the packages. To highlight the element of stronger ministerial and cross-agency collaboration, each priority also featured one or more "Wellbeing Approach in Action" narratives describing how different portfolio ministers were asked to work up initiative packages toward a common objective focused on the well-being outcomes signaled in the budget priorities.

For example, under the mental health priority—which was partly a response to outcome indicators showing that New Zealand's suicide rate for young people is among the worst in the OECD, with Māori and Pacific people particularly affected—packages of initiatives included increased frontline services, suicide prevention services, nurses in schools, and measures tackling homelessness, illustrating the cross-portfolio approach. One package focused particularly on mental health for offenders to break the cycle of reoffending involved the ministers of justice, corrections, and police working across their portfolios.

Under the priority for transforming the economy (to enable transition to a low-emissions economy, while supporting workers, businesses, and communities), a package of measures promoting productive and sustainable land use involved ministers for the environment, agriculture, climate change, research/science/innovation, conservation, land information, and forestry. The package included initiatives targeting the health of fresh waterways, New Zealand's climate change goals, and increased productivity of farmland.

The package responding to the priority relating to child well-being was notable as an example of the use of specific new legislative, governance, targeting, and reporting measures to support spending initiatives in the design of the government's intervention strategy. As a result of the Child Poverty Reduction Act 2018 (CPRA), the budget is now required to include a report on progress made in reducing child poverty measured against targets the government is required to set and publish, and on the impact of budget measures on child poverty. The Wellbeing Budget documentation duly included such reporting, including modeling of the impacts of earlier tax and welfare benefit system initiatives, some new income support initiatives in Budget 2019, and qualitative discussion of other measures the government viewed as relevant to the reduction of child poverty.

Development of the initiatives and packages involved some adaptation of existing assessment tools to align them with the LSF. The tools have always been focused on "value for money" and effective public financial management principles, and for some years those principles have explicitly taken a broad view of value and effectiveness, i.e., they have related explicitly to well-being outcomes. The tools include the Better Business Cases framework,[43] the *Guide to Social Cost-Benefit Analysis*,[44] and the CBAx spreadsheet model.

These tools facilitate comparison across initiatives and support analysts to develop their initiatives, including by providing common assumptions and outcome impact valuations, and by encouraging analysts to link the intervention logic underpinning their initiatives to the LSF outcome domains. The CBAx and CBA guidance emphasizes that monetization should be seen as an approach to comparing impacts in a common currency for outcomes that are inherently difficult to compare. The guidance recognizes the empirical and philosophical limits of such strategies and encourages pragmatism.[29,44] In that sense, the approach is similar to the use of Quality-Adjusted Life Years (QALYs), a relatively well-accepted means of comparing effect sizes in different domains of health.[45]

In other domains, such as environmental amenity, the lack of a common currency is quite evident, probably reflecting still limited understanding of complex ecological and biophysical processes. Reflecting such limits, the use of CBAx has generally been optional or limited to particular types of initiatives, to be used where an analyst views it as informative, depending on the inclination of the government at the time.

Examples of how departments used the CBAx tool in earlier budgets, and the kind of supporting well-being impact information they adduced to support their proposals, are on the Treasury's website.* Two detailed examples are the ones submitted by the Ministry of Education (2017)[46] for a proposal

* For examples from 2017, see *https://treasury.govt.nz/publications/information-release/applied-examples-cbax-budget-2017-information-release.*

to provide targeted and specialist support to 3- and 4-year-olds with oral language needs who are at risk for literacy difficulties, and by the Ministry of Justice (2017)[47] aiming to reduce youth offending among high-risk 14- to 16-year-olds by providing Cognitive Behavioral Therapy, Functional Family Therapy, and Professional Youth Mentoring services.

The CBAx tool user guidance is clear that quantitative modeling is just one part of CBA and policy analysis as applied to well-being. Policy decisions generally involve not just analysis (where the LSF plays an instrumental role), but also ministers judging alignment with a government's strategic priorities. As elected representatives, governments necessarily apply their own preference functions and value systems over the well-being domains as part of making resource allocation decisions. A well-being framework such as the LSF can help frame ministers' deliberations and bring the relevant evidence to bear more transparently and coherently.

Program and policy monitoring and evaluation

Using well-being frameworks to support policy monitoring and evaluation depends on sound evidence on the causal links from policy settings or interventions to well-being outcomes. The evidence is relevant to assessing current programs and services, reprioritization of spending across existing programs, or using existing funding to support new programs. The well-being outcomes of interest need to be distinguished from proxies or covariates, which might or might not have a causal role, and drivers and policy instruments.

As noted above, the government has given high profile to reducing child poverty, as one area in which well-being metrics and associated analysis are expected to be used to monitor progress and be used for accountability purposes:[33]

> An indicator of the direction of travel is the Prime Minister's Child Poverty Reduction Bill, not only setting agreed upon measures of child poverty, but also a requirement that each government [administration] set targets against those measures, and that governments report on child poverty indicators at every budget.

Previous governments in New Zealand have also used quantitative targets as part of the organization of public administration toward particular policy objectives. While these targets were not explicitly derived from or connected to LSF dimensions or measures, they served similarly to focus agencies on multi-agency outcome areas.[48] One such program, called Better Public Services, used targets explicitly as a device to organize public sector activity around ten high-profile, mostly social, outcome areas (such as reducing long-term welfare dependence, increasing participation in early childhood education, and increasing infant immunization rates), and to allow agencies and the government to be held to account for progress.

In the future, the budget bid templates and follow-through on implementation and evaluation will be further developed as part of ongoing efforts in New Zealand to improve the effectiveness of policy. However, there are both scientific and institutional challenges to meet. Evaluation of existing policy programs (particularly larger spending areas with possibly entrenched practices and worldviews) within a well-being framing, as a means to drive change, is one policy phase in which bureaucratic incentives, principal-agent problems, and other well-known issues can impede effective collective action. Public servants may be discouraged from thinking broadly if the management culture overemphasizes strict reporting with siloed lines of accountability and narrow output-based performance measures.[49,50] The challenge may be even more difficult if government systems and processes are complex and adaptive in the sense of Kurtz and Snowden (2003)[51] and Westley and Antadze (2010).[52] If the system impacts of interventions cannot be accurately predicted, an adaptive, learning-loop approach may be most likely to enable progress.

The large literature on policy coherence emphasizes the importance of avoiding institutional weaknesses, such as "layering" (failure to remove or adjust existing policy mechanisms before adding new ones), "drift" (changes to goals over time without changing the instruments, until the latter become poorly targeted to the goals), and "conversion" (attempting to adapt instruments designed for a particular goal to a new, unsuited goal).[53] These general issues of institutional discipline are not unique to well-being policy programs, of course. But to the extent that well-being approaches are expressly targeted to relatively complex and poorly understood policy problems, the issues are magnified. An attitude of humility, a strategy of adaptability, and a tactic of pragmatism in such a policy design environment are probably to be advised.

What Work Is Still Needed to Strengthen Government Well-Being Commitment and Practice?

Learning by doing, and the diffusion of well-being approaches across the system

The Treasury has signaled an intention to continue to develop the LSF while using it more broadly in day-to-day policy practice.[37] The learning gained is likely to influence most aspects of the LSF, including measurement and assessment tools and their use in government policy processes.

While the LSF work originated and continues to be housed within the Treasury, where it naturally fits with the agency's role in advising on the multi-faceted fiscal and economic aspects of the whole range of government activity, its location within a central ministry has also helped to embed the thinking and the tools consistently and coherently across government. The latter is necessary in light of the promise offered by the integration of aggregate and disaggregated well-being outcome frameworks over time. By such integration, one would hope that a common language can be developed to help simplify "wicked" (multi-outcome, multi-agency, multi-generational) problems to an analytically manageable state. Many such problems are social, involving individuals, families, or communities with complex needs that are typically poorly served by government agencies, even while those agencies produce relatively simple "main-stream" services to the bulk of the population efficiently and satisfactorily, on the whole, in New Zealand.[54]

In seeking to develop the LSF to support more effective well-being policy, the experiences with the development of the System of National Accounts (SNA, including GDP measurement) and Generally Accepted Accounting Principles (GAAP) for financial reporting are instructive. Both of these accounting systems were developed with a focus on particular applied policy purposes, and in the context of a clear demand from users for useable information.

Those accounting frameworks continue to serve New Zealand policymaking very well. In the case of the SNA, measurement of GDP and market income is needed for the purposes of measuring the tax revenue base and understanding macroeconomic dynamics at the aggregate national level. In the case of GAAP, credible and independent financial reporting has underpinned fiscal transparency and the soundness of government financial management and control. Both accounting systems are curated by internationally credible organizations. Both have evolved in response to their applied function, their users' needs, and improvements in the measurement technology, as all have also changed over time.

The need for awareness of limitations and further work

Users of any measurement or assessment framework need to be keenly aware of its limitations, and the challenge for the development of well-being frameworks is no different. Policymakers may expect too much from the frameworks in terms of their ability to guide policy precisely, given the limits of our knowledge in many important domains. What should be measured in order to assist policy, given the theory and user need, is as important as what can be measured. And the answers can only be fully revealed through using the frameworks in shaping policy, resource allocation, and program design.

The growing attention in many country settings and circumstances to aggregate well-being frameworks provides experience to learn from. Not only are national authorities and researchers pursuing initiatives, but subnational authorities are as well. This was assisted by legislative action in New Zealand in 2018, with a reform to local government legislation that reinstated the promotion of social, economic, environmental, and cultural well-being of communities to the statutory purpose of local governments. This provided some impetus to existing local and regional government initiatives in this area, with the Waikato Regional Council, for example, having published its Progress Indicators framework for a few years.[55] In New Zealand, civil society (e.g., the Salvation Army, Johnson [2018][56]) and business sector (e.g., Deloitte[57]) groups have also prepared their own well-being-oriented reports.

Usage of the LSF (or any other multidimensional outcomes framework) for the agenda-setting phase, which seeks to look across all areas of government activity, requires some ability to compare across all the dimensions measured. This is true at both the well-being domain level and at the level of all the disaggregated and derivative statistics (distributional statistics, subpopulation cuts, etc.) that are of interest to agenda-setters. As an analytical matter, this could include benchmarking against cross-country or historical reference levels or other norms, and conversion of the gaps into a common metric (for example, number of standard deviations).

Further work on alignment to develop common language, methods, and use of evidence would assist the well-being approach to mature, and this needs to be understood as a long-term strategy. Characterizing the capital stocks and measuring their direction of change is particularly challenging. Key choices also exist around which of the many possible distributional measures to focus on. The evolving practice with the child poverty targeting framework is likely to be instructive in this respect.

The capability approach and distributional elements of the LSF, as well as the diverse perspectives on well-being as revealed in the consultation and engagement conducted at various stages of its development, underscore the need for continued efforts to test the comprehensiveness and balance of the LSF in its application to various complex policy issues. Engagement with all the different perspectives on well-being can help to strengthen dialogue, participatory governance, and hence legitimacy. These in turn help to mitigate the risks of politicization and undermining of the durability of processes and analysis that can offer genuine and demonstrable value to the policy development process.

Recognition and hence better navigation of the distinction between the instrumental, conceptual/discursive, and political roles of well-being frameworks can also help.

In the nuts and bolts of proposal development, assessment, prioritization, and evaluation a massive analytical and evidential task remains to be surmounted. The key gap here is that the evidence base is very partial. Even where there may be good evidence on effect sizes and impacts, the studied outcome variables tend to be proximate to the interventions studied, rather than at the level of the well-being outcome domains in the LSF. This probably reflects the complexity and diffuseness of the causal chain between those outcome domains and the interventions available. A lot of judgment is therefore required to fill the gap. The socially constructed process of sense-making among government agencies and ministers as used in the government's Wellbeing Budget is an example of an early approach to bringing this necessary judgment to bear.

Considerable promise with new data and evidence

There is considerable promise in how well-being frameworks, such as the LSF, can help governments coherently address complex policy issues, both long-standing and emerging. A core strategic objective of the framework is to increase the positive influence of evidence on decisions. Nevertheless, ambition in well-being approaches needs to be tempered by an awareness of public sector capacity and capability, as well as the quality and comprehensiveness of the currently available data on well-being and lived experience. Here, at least some parts of the data ecosystem are growing rapidly. Rich longitudinal administrative datasets, such as New Zealand's Integrated Data Infrastructure,[58] enable longitudinal and highly granular views on subpopulations and may assist in enriching aggregate measures of well-being. Coupled with greater emphasis on evaluation and experimental design in the proposal stage, this will help strengthen the evidence base over time.

It should be clear from the above review of the use and intent of the LSF that, as a central agency–run aggregate framework that attempts to "cover everything," demonstrating positive impact from the framework comprehensively across the policy system is a somewhat daunting, long-term task. To help the well-being approach scale up and spread, aligned efforts from others will be essential. The ongoing development of the framework need not, and should not, preclude experimentation and smaller-scale or "grassroots" efforts at the level of individual government agencies, or indeed other actors, such as local community groups. The well-being outcomes framework can still provide a common language and a way of organizing the evidence and narratives about what such groups intend to achieve with their activities. Interventions implicitly targeting well-being can also be designed to generate evidence about their impact on well-being more clearly, to support potential scaling up.[59,60]

Conclusion

The Treasury's LSF is a coherent well-being framework, with a measurement taxonomy supported by clear theoretical and philosophical underpinnings. It has been developed and used in New Zealand as an integral part of the policy development and decision-making process to support central government policymaking, most recently in a core, high-profile government process, the annual budget.

The LSF is intended to address gaps in the way public policy addresses complex, multi-outcome, multi-agency, and multi-generational policy issues that involve substantial trade-offs and interdependencies. Many such issues are becoming more acute and urgent. Nevertheless, challenges to progress arise related to overcoming long-standing institutional processes and incentives encouraging siloed behavior and perspectives.

The framework plays a primarily instrumental role in helping to organize the evidence relevant for advice to governments about their well-being priorities. It recognizes that the diverse values and perspectives of the public, as expressed through the political process, are ultimately for ministers to respond to as elected representatives. The design of the framework and the approach is intended to underpin legitimacy and durability through political cycles, while also enabling the well-being evidence to better support decision-making, and ultimately better decisions.

The development and application of the framework has been pragmatic, attuned to function and the needs of users and informed by stakeholder engagement while also anchored to clear theoretical underpinnings. Policymakers are not necessarily especially interested in theorizing about, or measuring, well-being for their own sakes, but instead in tools and advice that can improve decision-making and accountability. Demonstrating the value, in terms of better policymaking, from measurement and "framework" efforts is both challenging and essential for building durable support within the official sector, among elected representatives and the general public.[59,60]

The public debate on the merits and usage of the LSF and well-being constructs more generally in New Zealand has been lively, especially since the government's announced intention to use it to inform its Wellbeing Budget— with not all of the commentary entirely positive (e.g., Dann [2018],[61] Grimes

[2017][62]). Some commentators appear to view the use of the well-being construct as a distraction from core economic and fiscal issues (e.g., Wilkinson [2016],[63] Reddell [2018][64]). Since the release of the Wellbeing Budget itself, commentators and analysts have shown keen interest in how the evidence base has been used to support the funded initiatives, and also in how the government intends to track and assess its progress against the budget priorities. The development of this discourse is encouraging, since it has the potential to support the focus of the public sector's and governments' attention on how to use the evidence best in the advice process.

New Zealand has attracted international attention from other countries for the Wellbeing Budget in particular, as the references from international media earlier in this chapter indicate. In international comparisons of the state of play in government well-being approaches, such as Exton & Shinwell (2018),[12] Durand (2018),[13] and Durand & Exton (2019),[10] New Zealand is counted as a country that has sought to drive well-being measurement through both policy advice processes and actual decision-making, which could be seen as a more ambitious undertaking than simply collating and reporting well-being measures.

The Treasury's pragmatic, emergent, and "learning by doing" approach reflects the early stages of understanding of how well-being frameworks can improve policy. Time and experience—in New Zealand and elsewhere—are needed to better understand the prevailing operating environment and space for change. Ambition is needed also, to drive momentum for institutionalizing what has already been achieved—tempered by an awareness of the risks of overburdening currently limited and partial technical knowledge. If the right balance can be struck, there is considerable potential for better government decisions and higher well-being for New Zealanders.

Opportunities Across Every Sector to Advance a Well-Being Framework

Discussion and Case Studies From Bellagio

Establishing well-being as a guiding construct for society ultimately requires a commitment across every sector and many fields, including health, education, technology, environment, and others. There are opportunities for exploration, programmatic and policy action, and leadership in the public, private, academic, and nonprofit environments, and opportunities for leaders and actors across these sectors to champion—through words and actions—this new way of looking at the world and making decisions.

Ideally, this work will happen in an interrelated and collaborative way that breaks down entrenched (and incentivized) habits of working in isolation. This is not a new idea, but as the group at Bellagio discussed, the well-being frame may facilitate cross-sector collaboration by resetting the goals—not around individual issues or functions, but around the much broader idea of creating the right conditions for current and future generations to thrive. These changes should be dynamic and shift over time, reflecting the "do, learn, inspire" cycle that some cities and countries as well as companies and NGOs are already trying. It encourages a culture that views failure as an opportunity for learning, and promotes incentives for experimentation in each sector and across sectors.

> *There are plenty of people doing siloed things; the space that's empty is the people who can tell the stories across the piece.*
>
> —*Carrie Exton*
> *Head of Section for Monitoring Well-Being and Progress*
> *Organisation for Economic Co-operation and Development*
> *France*

That said, there are also distinct roles and starting points within each sector, and the strategy for change may look different in every case. Because the group at

Bellagio represented most sectors, this was a lively discussion explored through the case studies, in small groups organized specifically by sector, and in the ongoing conversation about levers of change. This chapter outlines some potential actions within each sector and examples of learnings underway.

A Potential Starting Place for Inspiration and Innovation: International and Quasi-Governmental Organizations

A set of international bodies, such as the United Nations (UN), World Health Organization (WHO), and Organisation for Economic Co-operation and Development (OECD), are serving as catalysts for a well-being approach, often inspiring or even pushing governments and other sectors to innovate. There is opportunity to advance these groups' international standards that are already aligned with the well-being construct, and to integrate well-being indicators into other international standards, goals, and accords. As discussed in the previous chapter, New Zealand is an example of a country that has taken inspiration and source material from OECD's Better Life Index and applied it in the development of its Living Standards Framework and the nation's Wellbeing Budget.

Two other promising and aligned accords are the United Nations Sustainable Development Goals (SDGs) and the growing focus in investment and business certifications of Environmental, Social, and Governance (ESG) criteria. The SDGs are specific goals to end poverty, protect the planet, and ensure that all people enjoy peace and prosperity. In 2015, some 200 world leaders agreed to work toward meeting those goals by 2030. The SDGs are the result of a broad-based consensus and provide specific targets that governments, the social sector, and businesses can and are using to improve well-being for people around the world. While implementation has been uneven, some research has cited the influence of SDGs on other sectors. For example, a 2017 survey found that more than half of the impact investing industry is intent on tracking returns directly against SDG-related targets.[1] SDG 3, "Ensure healthy lives and promote well-being for all at all ages,"[2] is most directly aligned with a well-being approach. Tarek Abu Fakhr, adviser at the United Arab Emirates National Program for Happiness and Wellbeing, pointed out to Bellagio colleagues the need for this connection to be even more robust. "It's one thing to create a new narrative [about well-being], but it's another thing to push for our agenda and the well-being narrative to be included in something that is very high on the global agenda today, which is the SDGs," he said. "It's very unfortunate that well-being is only brought up in the context of mental health. We believe it has to be part of the bigger narrative."

The ultimate outcome of achieving the SDGs is actually people's well-being.
—*Tarek Abu Fakhr*
Adviser
National Program for Happiness and Wellbeing
United Arab Emirates

On the note of impact investing, application of ESG criteria in investment ratings, screenings, and considerations for investments by institutional investors are growing and are reaching far beyond impact investors to being increasingly mainstreamed. From the growth of the Global Impact Investing Rating System (GIIRS) and other investment ratings focused on ESG, to the CEO of BlackRock (one of the world's largest asset managers) predicting that all investors will use ESGs within five years,[3] the impacts of environmental, social, and governance considerations on business sustainability and success are gaining currency. Bellagio participant Shariha Khalid Erichsen, managing partner of global investment and impact advisory firm Mission & Co., noted that the environmental and governance domains in the ESG criteria are quite advanced, but the social criteria—how a company manages relationships with employees, suppliers, customers, and the communities where it operates—are not. A well-being approach could help advance those social criteria, including looking at the well-being of workers, supply chains, and other aspects. She noted that well-being impacts and measures could be of significant benefit to ESG-focused companies and that this private sector alignment could advance the use of a well-being framework more broadly.

These models have strong potential to inform efforts to advance a well-being framework at the national and local level, providing leadership, research-based guidance, connections between disparate work that is taking place across the world, and proof points to show government officials and private sector leaders how a well-being approach helps advance their goals. However, several cautionary notes also emerged: first, governments may sign off on metrics like the SDGs and publicly assert that they are using well-being metrics, while still carrying on with the same programs and policies, labeled differently, and not showing whether any change is actually occurring.

Second, although the SDGs provided opportunity for input and engagement during the development process more effectively than previous accords, attention is still needed to ensure a high level of community input—including voices that have typically been excluded—in the design of these models. One example participants raised was putting into practice the rights enumerated in the UN Declaration on the Rights of Indigenous Peoples, which was signed by 144 states in 2007. The UN Declaration establishes a universal framework of minimum standards for the survival, dignity, and well-being of the Indigenous peoples of the world, and it elaborates on existing human rights standards and fundamental freedoms as they apply to the specific situation of Indigenous peoples.

Third, international economic institutions, such as the International Monetary Fund, the World Bank, and OECD, need to continue to integrate well-being as a key dial on the dashboard and increasingly as a core outcomes goal for economic policy. These organizations and others must also increase dedicated resources that advance well-being, including tangible models of measurement, policies, practices, and approaches, as well as incentives for leaders to adopt and advance well-being outcomes. Bellagio participants noted that international development agencies, such as USAID, the Department for International Development (DFID) in the U.K., and others can be sources of funding for well-being efforts.

Because any international accord only makes a real difference if it is integrated into work taking place in specific nations, regions, and cities, it is also important to monitor actual implementation at the national level. Additionally, international measures should be continually assessed and modified as informed by local practice and success.

Civil Society: Opportunities to Innovate, Experiment, and Share Learning

Often the civil society sector—including nongovernmental organizations (NGOs), philanthropy, academia, and others—provides leadership in advocating for well-being approaches and piloting projects, which governments and other sectors then can help scale up. For example, in Palestine, Birzeit University's Institute of Community and Public Health has taken the lead in putting trauma in a broader context than the traditional individual, biomedical model. Its approach helps people understand their individual experience of trauma in collective, socio-political terms, which can be helpful in recovery.

The Institute's work has spurred partnerships in research on well-being with UNICEF and others, as well as work in the community with local NGOs, including a long-standing women's health program. The Palestinian Ministry of Health, meanwhile, has established a women's health directorate and program.

This reflects the flexibility and innovation possible in the nonprofit sphere, says Bellagio participant Gora Mboup, president and CEO of Global Observatory linking Research to Action (GORA) Corp in the United States and Senegal. "There are certain NGOs who have moved away from GDP itself and have developed what they call a basic needs questionnaire," he said. "And they implement it at the local level. They do not implement it at the national level. They will go to a community and list not only the basic-needs ranking but also what can they do and what they are doing."

As an example, Engage Nova Scotia is an independent NGO supported through funding from the public, private, community, and academic sectors. It is building a new measurement framework that incorporates the views of Nova Scotians to redefine and rediscover what success means. The initiative's Advisory Group and key partners are made up of advocates from environment, industry, poverty reduction, sports, academia, government, and community groups. The role of the provincial government is as a supporter and partial funder, but not as the leader. The goal, shared Danny Graham, CEO at Engage Nova Scotia, with his fellow Bellagio participants was to reduce the risk of the initiative becoming a political football during election cycles, and also to allow for nimbleness and leadership from a coalition of trusted partners.

Social movements may also be allies in advancing a well-being framework from within the civil sector. The idea of prioritizing well-being as an outcome of policies and practices has much in common with efforts to advance human rights, economic equity, environmental justice, sustainable development goals, quality of life, livable cities, healthy cities, inclusive cities, prosperous cities, sustainability, and resilience, among others. Aligning and collaborating with these movements would enable advocates of a well-being framework to share information and expertise about potential allies, engagement strategies, narratives, advocacy tactics, and opportunities for influence. It would build the network of people and organizations prepared to respond to threats and opportunities, and would build greater currency for emerging well-being narratives and approaches.

> *I'm curious about how well-being connects to social movements. I'm curious whether the idea of well-being allows us to unravel the criminal justice system and to re-create it in a different form, whether it allows us to create relationships around gender, and race, and class, and ethnicity, and religion, and sexuality in new and different ways. And I'm curious about how this might completely re-imagine our relationship to the environment.*
>
> —*Mallika Dutt*
> *Founder and Director*
> *Inter-Connected*
> *United States*

Engaging funders to advance well-being approaches

The philanthropy sector—including private, corporate, family, religious, and high-net-worth individuals—is a vital partner to fund research and innovation, seed promising approaches and help bring them to scale, and make important contributions in ways that government bodies alone cannot.

"There are some philanthropies that are focused on health, some that focus on justice, some that focus on education, but together they are all dealing with different upstream drivers of well-being," said Bellagio participant Anita Chandra, vice president and director for RAND Social and Economic Well-Being. "Perhaps they can give a half a billion dollars each year, but together there is some forced amplification to ultimately impact these well-being outcomes."

> *There is the potential [for philanthropies] to fund together with a longer lens.*
> —*Anita Chandra*
> *Vice President and Director*
> *RAND Social and Economic Well-Being*
> *RAND Corporation*
> *United States*

Participants mentioned that some foundations are increasingly looking for experiments—including those that fail—to demonstrate social impact and share best practices, and encouraged much more of this. In particular, there is a need and opportunity to catalogue and scale up examples of "positive deviancy," places where there are rising levels of well-being despite objectively challenging conditions, lack of homogeneity, or other factors. Bellagio participant Claire Nelson, lead futurist of the Futures Forum in the United States and the Caribbean, encouraged funders to be open to ideas packaged in unconventional ways from people outside their usual circles. Radical thinkers, sometimes less likely to receive funding, may be precisely the innovators whose ideas can provide new insights into supporting a well-being framework, she said.

Working with businesses

Participants noted that there are many entry points to working with businesses on adopting a well-being framework. Among them are with executives who already believe in such an approach and can help spread it through their practices, policies, and thought leadership. In fact, in recent years, over 50,000 businesses have taken the B Impact Assessment (one of the most rigorous sets of international standards for social, environmental, workplace, governance, and community responsibility); over 3,000 businesses in 64 countries have met the level required to be certified as B Corporations. In order to quickly reach business leaders, participants suggested tapping into this and other existing forums that many CEOs participate in, such as Davos (the World Economic Forum), the Skoll World Forum, and other global networks.

And it is important to speak the language of business, they said. Bellagio participant Kee-Seng Chia said that the Saw Swee Hock School of Public Health at the National University of Singapore, where he is founding dean, made successful inroads with businesses by highlighting the cost of diabetes among the working population. They showed that in 2010, there were 180,000 people with diabetes in the working population, which cost Singapore $1 billion. The idea was to get the message across that chronic diseases, not just workplace accidents, have a tremendous impact on the bottom line.

> *Money talks, and to change policy with employers, with corporations, with government we have to talk dollars and cents.*
>
> —*Kee-Seng Chia*
> *Founding Dean and Professor*
> *Saw Swee Hock School of Public Health*
> *National University of Singapore*

Well-being advocates are also looking for ways to influence the next generation of business leaders. The group discussed economics programs at universities around the world where students are challenging the traditional paradigms and advancing more holistic models. RWJF funded a collaboration between Harvard's Business School and School of Public Health to create a business curriculum case for a Culture of Health,* which has strong parallels with a well-being framework, Alonzo Plough, chief science officer and vice president of the Robert Wood Johnson Foundation, noted to Bellagio participants.

"The business folks reframed our framework in a way where the core concepts were the same but it's very business friendly in its constructs," Plough noted. "I think we have to be very flexible with our constructs—not our core values but our constructs—so we can engage with other sectors."

Businesses, foundations, and NGOs will need simple tools and decision-making aids as well as case studies and other examples of how the idea of using well-being as a core measure of progress is being translated into practice. Model legislation, policies, and programs—as well as insights into how they played out in cities, communities, and countries—will also help companies and nonprofits track what works and what does not. Participants noted a number of examples that advocates can draw from; for instance, the clothing company Eileen Fisher has adopted a stronger well-being focus, in part through its work with the GNH Centre Bhutan.

---

* The Culture of Health for Business Framework received a 2020 World Changing Ideas Award from Fast Company: *https://www.fastcompany.com/90492149/world-changing-ideas-awards-2020-corporate-social-responsibility-finalists-and-honorable-mentions*

Bellagio participant Nancy Wildfeir-Field noted that the organization she leads, GBCHealth, is a coalition of businesses committed to investing their resources to make a healthier world for their employers, communities, and the larger world. She said that she welcomed the opportunity to both collaborate and use its platform to move the well-being approach forward. "I want to start thinking about how I can help companies more clearly integrate this into their discussions and their strategies," she said.

> [Integrating a well-being approach in business] is actually much more than just their CSR strategy. It really is about integration into workplace policies, interaction with governments, et cetera.
>
> —Nancy Wildfeir-Field
> President
> GBCHealth
> United States and Africa

The business sector can also be an investor in well-being efforts. One example is hybrid models, such as cooperatives, some of which are quite large, that apply market-based solutions to increasing economic livelihoods and are pushing forward an agenda for the people they represent. Erichsen described Mondragon Cooperative Corporation, a federation of more than 200 worker cooperatives based in the Basque region of Spain that employs over 78,000 people and has revenues of almost 13 billion euros a year. At the other end of the spectrum, she said, Sahyadri is a farmers' group in India that is self-organizing to provide microfinance. Erichsen also pointed to peer-to-peer fundraising platforms that use technology to provide access to loans; these are among the fastest-growing industries in the finance space. While these particular models are separate from well-being theory, economic stability is part of people's well-being, making strategies like this a potential component of broad efforts to advance a well-being approach.

Another potential avenue for investing in well-being efforts is sovereign wealth funds, which are state-owned investment funds derived from a country's reserves to benefit the country's economy and citizens. Finally, participants felt that social impact bonds might be an option, though these are considered risky investments because they only pay investors if social outcomes and savings are achieved.

Well-Being Approaches in Government: Opportunities for Integration

Governments that have adopted a well-being framework have been influenced by both larger shifts in the world, such as the SDGs and OECD's well-being work, as well as their own internal pressures and opportunities. Some turn to it for new solutions to persistent problems, or in the face of a recession or other crisis, realizing that the old way of doing things is not working. On a more cynical note, Bellagio participants said, others may be swept up in the competitive urge to rank within the happiest countries as international rankings gain currency, or may use it as a way to push responsibility onto the citizens, implying that the reason things are not going well is because people aren't connected, not because the government has failed in budget and policy.

Some of the most visible examples of governments adopting a well-being framework are at the national level, driven by leaders with an interest in and commitment to improving well-being, and often in countries that are smaller, more homogenous, and where an existing commitment to participatory dialogue with citizens already exists. Less visible but often highly effective are the well-being framework efforts happening at the more nimble local level; there is great opportunity, participants stressed, to learn from and scale up these innovative approaches.

When governments decide to integrate well-being indicators deliberately into their policies, they have typically used five key mechanisms, according to Carrie Exton, a Bellagio participant, and head of OECD's Section for Monitoring Well-Being and Progress, and Martine Durand, also of OECD.[4] Those mechanisms are: (1) budgeting decisions (allocation of public spending to broaden decision-making beyond GDP); (2) legislation (passing laws to secure long-term change in government policy); (3) strategic planning and performance frameworks (a method to set out priorities for national progress in the medium and long term); (4) creating new institutional structures or positions to promote well-being, such as new ministry positions, government departments, or accountability mechanisms; and (5) providing capacity building and guidance for civil servants (e.g., training on translating a well-being framework into actual policy and practice).

A key message from the Bellagio gathering was that *how* that work should take place will be different depending on the context, particularly in where leadership lies. There was wide agreement that government approaches will be most successful when coordination and collaboration are baked into the model, recognizing that solutions to complex issues cannot come from one department or funding stream alone.

There are examples of this idea in action in Bhutan, Singapore, and the United Arab Emirates (UAE), among other places, that have deliberately ensured that efforts to improve well-being have not become a vertical responsibility but rather integrated throughout government agencies. For example, the UAE government decided not to have a stand-alone Ministry of Happiness and Wellbeing, but instead appointed a Minister of Happiness and Wellbeing who sits within the prime minister's office. This minister has direct access to the central government and oversight over ministries accountable for this work. Additionally, the government linked its priority on happiness to measurable actions across systems.

Abu Fakhr provided an example of how this central leadership, collaborating across the government, has led to early-stage action in the UAE. The government conducted a national survey on happiness and well-being and found that 40 percent of a person's well-being has to do with their family. It also found that one-third of the working population is not happy with their work-life balance, and that just 2 percent of schoolchildren spent time with their fathers during the school week.

In response, the UAE implemented a new national back-to-school policy. All federal government employees would have three hours of free time on the first day of school—or three hours per day for a full week for parents with children in kindergarten—to take their children or pick them up from school. A number of local government entities and private sector employers also adopted that policy.

"This holistic approach to happiness and well-being allowed for cross-sectoral insights that would otherwise not be possible," Abu Fakhr said. "It resulted in bringing together student well-being from the education sector, family connectedness from social development, and work-life balance from labor, all under one policy."

In Bhutan the well-being approach is being operationalized at a country level, through collaboration among different entities that have evolved to play distinct, but complementary roles—linking research, government, and civil society. The Center for Bhutan Studies and GNH Research, an autonomous social science research institute, conducts and analyzes a national GNH survey, alongside other research initiatives. The GNH Commission, a government planning body, applies a GNH screening tool to assess policies and projects through a well-being lens, and integrates GNH within the country's 5-year development plans. The GNH Centre Bhutan, a national civil society organization, aims to translate GNH into practical action at the grassroots level, through outreach and collaboration with key sectors, and through GNH leadership and action-learning programs in Bhutan and internationally.

For governments just getting started in well-being approaches, participants pointed out that there are opportunities to bring a well-being focus into policies during times like budgeting and other moments when people come together within and across agencies to make choices and decisions. Those places of convergence create an opening for well-being approaches to spread. Exton pointed out that many policymakers already view themselves as investing significantly in their constituents' well-being based on the relative amounts of resources budgeted for health, education, environment, and other services compared to the amounts budgeted for commerce and economic development. Meeting these leaders where they are and focusing on *redefining* growth or progress around well-being (versus becoming locked in debate over the extent to which GDP is the "right" indicator) can create an opportunity to build allies. Additionally, Danny Graham noted the importance of meeting consistently with opposition leaders and getting their input and buy-in, in part to build durability in this work that can last even when government leaders change.

Working at Different Levels of Government

Specific considerations and opportunities exist at local, regional, and national levels of government to advance a well-being framework. And all levels of government can create synergies by working together and making use of each of their particular strengths and positions. For example, effective local actions can be lifted up to replicate and scale nationally, while national and international measurement insights can be useful to local communities embarking on change. Central government, said participants, needs to ask what it can do to be helpful (and not a barrier) on the ground, and to learn from and scale up the disruptive change happening at the local level.

> *"Local itself is good. But it doesn't pursue policy change for the whole system. But a whole system approach without creating a connection with the local is too much top down and would probably affect having a shared vision."*
> —*José Molinas Vega*
> *Minister-Secretary of Planning for Economic and*
> *Social Development*
> *Republic of Paraguay*

Local

A clear theme running through the Bellagio conference was the need to listen to and act on what people need, what matters to them and how *they* define well-being. Local communities (which in the Bellagio discussions included towns and cities as well as states and provinces) can bring in regional, national, or even international well-being frameworks, but these must be viewed as a starting point to consider and adapt. (See chapter 8 for more on grassroots engagement in defining and implementing a well-being approach.)

Well-being and happiness is so personal, and a lot of the work we're trying to do is at the national and international level. At the end of the day, it boils down to how the person experiences his or her well-being and happiness locally.

—Shariha Khalid Erichsen
Managing Partner
Mission & Co.
Southeast Asia

David Bornstein, co-founder and CEO of Solutions Journalism Network in the United States, pointed out to fellow Bellagio participants that when people across the United States have conversations about what should happen in their community, the core of these questions is: will it contribute to economic growth? But these questions do not take place in a framework where people can evaluate competing interests or look at decisions through a lens of well-being, Bornstein noted.

"So what I get really excited about is this: what would happen if this [well-being] framework with simple decision aids were put in the hands of town councils where when people want to make a decision about something really basic to the local environment . . . such as do we need a better transportation system, should we fund transport for the elderly—these are real decisions that happen every day—people can have these conversations, and they could have a framework," Bornstein said.

He continued, "I've seen many conversations around the United States where it's really clear that people are relying on the testimony of a few experts [for decisions] like whether or not a Walmart would be good for the town. And they're really not considering many, many things. Even just to test [a well-being lens] with a few dozen communities and see: Does it change the conversation? Does it change the kind of decisions people make? Does it make people feel like they had more to say or more power in the future of their town and shaping it? I think it's really an enormously powerful framework."

Participants also stressed the need to create environments where it's possible to "try 100 things," such as the Health in Our Hands movement. That is, start with simple changes that have a tangible effect, measure the change to see what works, and share the data to learn from it and spread successes to other communities. They dubbed this "radical experimentation" and noted that organizations like the International Association of Community Development are undertaking such work in some 150 countries.

Liz Zeidler also noted to fellow Bellagio participants that starting locally makes sense because "local is where people experience their well-being and are interested in the well-being of their local places. It is also where a lot of innovation is happening. It's going to take a long time to get to a global accord on an alternative to the GDP, so let's get on with it locally." Her U.K. organization, Happy City, where she is chief executive, works with city and municipal governments to put "thriving lives" at the heart of their decision-making. Happy City does that in part by offering measurement tools, including the Thriving Places Index, that provide a framework for evaluating and reporting well-being at the local levels. It has published the Thriving Places Index results for 373 local authorities in England and Wales and is currently working with 12 of those authorities to embed this framework into their operations.

National

At the national level, a key theme was the importance of creating a national story or identity of well-being. That is, getting away from a narrative about "we're known for producing the most [of something]" to "we're known for having a great quality of life, people are happy here, and here's what that means."

To help create a national well-being ethos in which different sectors come together in a shared narrative, some ministries and government agencies are actively collaborating in areas like agenda setting, resource allocation, and even how they define problems. For example, instead of saying that an agency works on housing, it might say it works on livability, which incorporates far more than physical structures and zoning, and also incorporates social connection, community supports, ownership supports, etc. By definition, this agency would have to work across government functions, breaking down silos and taking a more holistic approach.

As discussed in the previous chapter, in New Zealand, the national Treasury developed the Living Standards Framework (LSF) as a tool to improve its policy advice and strategic thinking on intergenerational well-being. Tim Ng, deputy secretary and chief economic adviser of the New Zealand Treasury, noted at Bellagio that the LSF has always been envisioned as a practical tool that will allow Treasury analysts to develop a common language at the central level to create and use a well-being framework to inform policy and resource allocation. Ng noted that one of the benefits of taking this approach is that it helps in deciding questions of public policy around intergenerational well-being.

"Politicians repeatedly say—and it plays well with the public—that we're here to preserve things for our children, making things better for our future generations, and so on," Ng said. "But then through the political process you can actually end up with a whole lot of policies and spending initiatives that unduly favor the current generation at the expense of future generations."

If you really are serious about future generations, then you need to recognize the trade-off between drawing down capitals to fund initiatives for the current population at the expense of future populations.

—Tim Ng
Deputy Secretary and Chief Economic Adviser
The New Zealand Treasury

The three devolved legislatures of the United Kingdom—Scotland, Wales, and Northern Ireland—have undertaken a deliberate approach to reframe the role of government as one that seeks to improve societal well-being, in part out of frustration in seeing little progress in improving outcomes over the years.[5] Those jurisdictions have implemented new public policy reforms as well as frameworks to measure progress on reaching their goals. These governments also had some characteristics that align with a well-being approach: they all have relatively small populations, close relationships between parts of the government system that may have helped in coming to a shared belief in the importance of addressing the problem, and mechanisms that either encourage or require cross-party collaboration. Those governments, which are geographically close and bound together by a common language and central government also, to some extent, influenced one another in their work. Scotland, for example, was the first government in the area to take on a well-being approach; its example and successes then encouraged Northern Ireland government officials to take similar actions.

Specific to Scotland's approach, in 2011, some 800 people came together to create what became a vision to make the country the best place in the world for children to grow up. To make this vision a reality, Bellagio participant Sir Harry Burns, professor of global public health at the University of Strathclyde and Scotland's former chief medical officer, noted that the leaders of the Early Years Collaborative, a multi-agency collaboration including social services, health, education, police, and nongovernmental agencies, decided that they wanted to reduce the stillbirth rate by 15 percent by 2015. They also set targets for developmental progress at age 30 months.

If you want change to happen you have to be able to write down what you want to change, by how much, by when, and by what method.

—Harry Burns
Professor, Global Public Health
University of Strathclyde
Scotland

Finally, national governments can play a role in shifting measurement and reporting to use well-being indicators. One suggestion offered by participants was that governments focus on impact at the highest level (e.g., reduction in war and violence, increase in economic equity) versus merely tracking changes in systems and structures, then make the causal link between a well-being approach and that impact.

Conclusion

A clear takeaway from the Bellagio meeting is that making an impact on well-being can start in any sector and at any level, responding to specific needs, and that efforts become even more powerful when sectors begin working together. What seems to help propel those collaborations is when they provide a neutral platform where people from each sector bring both their own expertise *and* an openness and willingness to try something new, outside of the regular thinking and ways of doing business. Outside urgency and pressure, such as the SDGs or concerns about the environment, also seem to be an important spur to multiple sectors acting both on their own and together.

As these collaborations grow—across the private sector, across government ministries, and between these and other sectors—the benefits of closer alignment and shared agendas become apparent. Among them, says Ng, is the ability for governments to share information about good practices with businesses that might be interested in taking a well-being lens to their work, and for unanticipated partnerships to take place between organizations that would not have connected otherwise. Closer collaboration can also lead to stronger networks of people and groups that can better manage threats such as rapidly emerging communicable diseases.

The group identified opportunities for leaders and organizations to plug into existing collaborations and co-creation efforts that are aligned with a well-being approach, such as the SDGs, ESGs, and the Open Government Partnership (a worldwide coalition of government leaders and civil society advocates that works to promote accountable, responsive, and inclusive governance). In addition, there are emerging cross-sector initiatives focused on sharing information and learnings to advance a well-being approach, including the Wellbeing Economy Alliance (WEAll) and Wellbeing Economy Governments partnership (WEGo), represented at Bellagio by Katherine Trebeck, knowledge and policy lead for the global Wellbeing Economy Alliance.

"What we're really after is the common good," said Bellagio participant Jennifer Prah Ruger, Amartya Sen professor of health equity, economics and policy at the University of Pennsylvania, "and the sense of connectedness that we all have with each other, that we have with nature, and our collective energy and enterprise to do more than we can do individually."

CASE STUDIES

World Tour of Well-Being in Action

Well-being approaches vary widely depending on cultural context, leadership, public interest, government structure, strength of civil society, and many other factors. This is why having practitioners—representing very diverse contexts and approaches from different parts of the world—at Bellagio was so vital to getting out of the theoretical and academic and onto the ground.

As they shared their experiences, it became clear that there is no magic formula. What works in Palestine is very different than what works in Bristol, United Kingdom, and is wholly dependent on what well-being means to people in those contexts. Nova Scotia and Singapore are both interested in a new narrative, but the story they will tell about well-being and the narrative they are seeking to shift looks as different as the skylines of these two places.

Cited throughout the chapters, the case studies shared at Bellagio appear here in their entirety. Some represent well-established efforts while others are just getting started. Some address well-being across many strategies; others are starting with an aspect, such as narrative change. They span hemispheres, include some places that are quite homogenous and some that are anything but. They consider a wide range of economic, social, cultural, political, and environmental contexts, and introduce us to how well-being approaches look in times of peace and times of war. Within each are insights, lessons, and even cautions that are relevant around the world. Recognizing and respecting the expertise and experience of the practitioners, each case is told from the perspective of the Bellagio participant from that area; specific insights or political nuance are their own, not those of the Robert Wood Johnson Foundation.

Mirroring how this book is organized, each case study explores: how well-being is defined in the country; how local narrative and culture support an enabling environment for success; grassroots engagement and shifts in power dynamics in favor of societal well-being; and key players working in tandem to advance the work. Each case study concludes with an overview of results from activities to date, instructive insights for others interested in a well-being approach, and a glimpse into where efforts in that region are anticipated to go next.

We hope these stories serve to inspire thinking about the diverse well-being approaches governments, civil society, and research institutions are taking around the world, and that these examples will encourage you to consider how well-being approaches may be best adapted for the context where you live and work.

Case Study From Bhutan

In Pursuit of Gross National Happiness

Based on contributions at the Bellagio convening from
Julia Kim, Program Director,
GNH Centre Bhutan

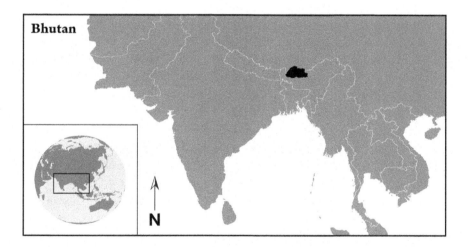

Introduction

The term "Gross National Happiness" or GNH emerged in the 1970s, when journalists asked Bhutan's Fourth King about his country's gross national product. The young king's reply, that "Gross National Happiness is more important than gross national product," clearly articulated his vision that the happiness and well-being of the country, rather than simply its economic output, should be the focus of the country's development.

Over time, key aspects for operationalizing the GNH vision as a development framework have been articulated and formalized. Four pillars of GNH were identified in 1998 (sustainable and equitable socioeconomic development, environmental conservation, preservation and promotion of culture, and good governance), followed by nine GNH "domains," which are now monitored through a national GNH survey. The Fourth King subsequently oversaw a peaceful transition to a constitutional monarchy, with the country's first democratic elections being held in 2008. GNH continues to hold central importance within the country's Constitution, which proclaims: "The State shall strive to promote those conditions that will enable the pursuit of Gross National Happiness."

Context Snapshot

- Leadership: GNH efforts are, and have been since their founding, spearheaded by the country's leaders, and have strong cultural and historical roots. Today, a range of organizations aim to support the government to realize this vision, including the GNH Commission, the Centre for Bhutan Studies and GNH Research, and the GNH Centre Bhutan.
- Stage of change: This work is among the most mature of all examples of a well-being approach. First articulated as "GNH" in the 1970s, happiness and well-being have remained a focus for the government ever since. Current opportunities and challenges include deepening awareness and engagement around GNH in Bhutan as the country continues to modernize, and adapting GNH values and metrics to other contexts and countries.
- Emphasis: Bhutan began with a clear vision from the leadership, and since 2008 has been using measurement to inform policy and practice. This is undertaken through national GNH surveys, the application of a GNH policy screening tool, and integration of GNH within the country's five-year development plans.

Defining and Measuring Well-Being

As former Prime Minister Jigme Y. Thinley has noted, the meaning of GNH needs to be distinguished from the fleeting, pleasurable moods often associated with the term "happiness." Instead, GNH refers to "the deep, abiding happiness that comes from living life in full harmony with the natural world, with our communities and fellow beings, and with our culture and spiritual heritage—in short, from feeling totally connected with our world." This concept of well-being suggests a "higher purpose" for development, including the realization of individual and collective human potential, in balance with the natural world.

In Bhutan, the role of government is regarded as creating the "enabling conditions" for happiness and well-being, which are defined and measured through the nine domains of the GNH Index:

- Psychological well-being
- Health
- Education
- Time use
- Cultural diversity and resilience
- Good governance
- Community vitality
- Ecological diversity and resilience
- Living standards

To assess changes in the nine domains over time, the Centre for Bhutan Studies (CBS) and GNH Research administer a national, population-based GNH survey, which includes 33 indicators and 124 variables. A threshold level is used to assess sufficiency within the 33 indicators, and overall, an individual experiencing sufficiency in six or more of the nine domains is considered "happy"—that is, to have sufficient conditions for happiness. Disaggregating data from the survey allows for comparisons across different groups, e.g., by age, gender, educational level, occupation, or geographic district.

In order to align government decision-making with GNH, the GNH Commission (a government planning body) uses a GNH policy-screening tool to provide a systematic appraisal of the potential effects of proposed projects on the nine domains. A policy that fails to receive a sufficiently high score is not necessarily rejected, but is sent back to the proponent agency, outlining why it fell short along with ways to improve it. The GNH Index can also be used to guide resource allocation and policy priorities, and since 2008, targets in the country's five-year plans are based on components of the Index.

Cultural Narrative

The government's role in creating happiness (*dekid*) for the people was acknowledged as far back as the legal code of 1729, which states that "If a government cannot create happiness for the people, there is no reason for government to exist." The context for a common well-being narrative in Bhutan has also been influenced by the Buddhist notion of a "Middle Path," based on avoiding extremes, living with moderation, and balancing both the material and intangible conditions for well-being (as reflected in the nine domains). These domains are regarded as being interdependent—a holistic view that does not privilege economic factors above others, but places them alongside a range of social and environmental concerns. Moreover, the well-being of human beings is regarded as intimately interconnected with that of the natural world—thus GNH expresses an "eco-centric" rather than "ego-centric" worldview, one in which balance and harmony among living systems are seen as integral.

Grassroots Engagement and Shifting Power to Build Equity

Historically, Bhutan has benefited from the influence of visionary leaders, such as the Fourth King, who have inspired and driven national GNH efforts. As the country has transitioned to a constitutional monarchy, the presence and activity of civil society organizations (CSOs) has begun to expand, and with it, their role in grassroots engagement around GNH. Many such organizations would not necessarily view themselves as "GNH organizations," yet are actively engaged in creating the enabling conditions for well-being—through improving equity and access across a range of key areas, including access to health services, housing and living standards, literacy, gender, media and communication, entrepreneurship, and job skills training. The national GNH survey is intended to highlight those groups that fall below the sufficiency level for well-being, and to identify which domains need to be strengthened. By doing so, inequities can be addressed, whether through government initiatives or through civil society actors and others at the grassroots level.

Collaboration Among Government, Civil Society, and Research

In order to operationalize the vision of GNH at a country level, collaboration among different bodies and stakeholders is required. In Bhutan, the following three entities have evolved to play distinct, but complementary, roles linking government, civil society, and research:

- The GNH Commission, a government body that applies the GNH "screening tool" in order to assess policies and projects through a GNH lens, and which integrates GNH within the country's five-year development plans.
- The Center for Bhutan Studies and GNH Research, an autonomous social science research institute established by the government of Bhutan, which conducts and analyzes the national GNH survey, alongside other research initiatives.
- The GNH Centre Bhutan, a national civil society organization that aims to translate GNH into practical action at the grassroots level, through outreach and collaboration with key sectors, and through GNH leadership and action-learning programs in Bhutan and internationally.

Results

Bhutan has conducted three rounds of GNH surveys, starting with a pilot survey in 2006, and nationwide surveys in 2010 and 2015. Guided by the GNH philosophy, the country has introduced a range of policies to achieve sustainable and equitable development while preserving its cultural traditions. Recent priorities have included poverty reduction, universal primary school enrollment, free access to basic health services, distribution of land to land-less farmers, expanded public services and infrastructure in rural areas, and increasing women's participation in elected office. There have been significant improvements in key social indicators, including a reduction in poverty and infant mortality rates, rising life expectancy, and substantial increases in primary school enrollment.

On the environmental front, Bhutan's Constitution commits to maintain a "minimum of 60 percent of the country's total land under forest cover for all time"; and the country has garnered recent attention as the world's first carbon-negative country—keeping greenhouse gas emissions well below its sequestration capacity. Other notable initiatives include the striking absence of outdoor advertising due to a ban on billboards, as well as Bhutan's "high value, low impact" tourism policy, which seeks to balance the income derived from its considerable tourism appeal, against potentially negative environmental and social impacts.

Recognizing the importance of integrating GNH principles within the country's schools, the Ministry of Education has been implementing a nationwide Educating for GNH initiative since 2010. Further efforts are underway to update and strengthen these initial curricula and training approaches. Recognizing the importance of aligning GNH principles and metrics within the country's emerging private sector, the Centre for Bhutan Studies and GNH

Research recently piloted a new GNH survey tool designed for guiding business development in Bhutan.

On a global level, Bhutan has contributed to a range of international initiatives that have brought growing attention to the importance of well-being and "beyond GDP" measures. In 2011, under Bhutan's leadership, the UN General Assembly adopted by consensus UN Resolution 65/309, "Happiness: Towards a holistic approach to development." The following year, the Royal Government of Bhutan convened a High-Level Meeting on Well-Being and Happiness: Defining a New Economic Paradigm. More than 800 participants, including political leaders, civil society organizations, media, and business, as well as leading economists, environmental activists, academics, and spiritual leaders joined the gathering. The following year, a final report highlighting key implications and recommendations for the international community was submitted to the UN General Assembly.

In the wake of this domestic and international experience, there has been growing interest in applying and adapting GNH values and approaches across a range of countries and contexts. Responding to this interest, in 2013 the GNH Centre Bhutan, together with the Global Leadership Academy (GIZ/ BMZ, Germany), and the Presencing Institute (Cambridge, USA) co-founded the "The Global Wellbeing Lab: Transforming Economy and Society." The Lab is a multi-stakeholder action-learning platform that aims to advance new ways of generating and measuring well-being at multiple levels of society. In addition, the GNH Centre has collaborated with Schumacher College (United Kingdom) and others to launch a series of courses (e.g., the Right Livelihood Program and the GNH Practitioner Program), which aim to re-align the values of work and economy toward greater well-being and a more sustainable society. By combining transformative leadership development (vision and values) with practical action (well-being innovation and prototypes), these initiatives are generating new lessons regarding how well-being concepts can be applied and adapted across a range of contexts, at individual and organizational levels.

Instructive Insights for Others Pursuing a Well-Being Approach

Commit to a multi-level, multi-sector approach. Bhutan has uniquely benefited from leaders who have articulated a national development strategy based on happiness and well-being. As this small Himalayan country, bordered by China and India, continues to chart an alternative course against the tide of conventional GDP-based development, the journey ahead will undoubtedly be challenging. What is clear, however, is that the steps Bhutan has taken to integrate and operationalize a GNH approach (articulating the vision within key legal instruments, such as the Constitution, developing and applying new survey and policymaking tools, and engaging influential sectors of society) are instrumental in taking a well-being approach beyond vision and into action. This multi-level, multi-sector approach can provide useful insights for other countries embarking on a similar course.

Start where you are, introducing well-being approaches across diverse scales and contexts. While a national-level approach may not initially be feasible in many countries, it is possible to introduce well-being metrics and approaches at a smaller scale, where innovation and learning can progress in a supportive environment. Through its action-learning platforms, the GNH Centre Bhutan has supported stakeholders from a range of countries to introduce well-being metrics and values at different levels of society (e.g., municipality, city, organization), as well as across key sectors of influence (e.g., business, education, city planning, health, social enterprise). As such initiatives grow over time, they can generate practical leverage points and popular support for subsequently mainstreaming new progress measures at a wider, systemic level. In this way, a *culture of equity and well-being* can be grown from the grassroots level, so that there is fertile soil for the seeds of new national level well-being measures and policies to land.

Go beyond numbers to transformative leadership for a unifying narrative of well-being. New progress indicators and measures are critical in shifting national priorities and budgets toward promoting greater well-being and equity. But numbers alone are not enough. Experience has shown that in the absence of deeply internalized values, reporting on measurements can remain an intellectual exercise, open to misinterpretation or manipulation in service of political agendas. For this reason, *transformative leadership development* forms a central part of the GNH Centre's programs, and in this context, participants have found it revealing to apply a "GNH lens" to their own personal lives. Demystifying economics and reconnecting it to ecology, well-being, and everyday lived experience is vital in revealing the deeper meaning behind the numbers. Participants can then begin to explore how a *unifying narrative of well-being* is supported by the growing research documenting how inequality negatively impacts not only the well-being of the poor, but also the privileged within society. This in turn shifts the level of inquiry from a position of fear, to one of curiosity and hope—not simply asking *what do we stand to lose*, but what do we stand to *gain* by shifting the current system?

The Road Ahead

Bhutanese citizens are often surprised and somewhat taken aback to find themselves the subject of such keen interest by the international community. For visitors, the inclination to paint Bhutan with an exotic "Shangri-la" brush is all too tempting and can sometimes project unrealistic expectations on this modest country that has chosen to embark on a unique development path. In the words of the first prime minister of Bhutan, "Bhutan is not a country that has attained GNH. Like most developing nations, we are struggling with the challenge of fulfilling the basic needs of our people. What separates us, however, from most others is that we have made happiness—the foundation of human needs—as the goal of social change."

From the inclusion of happiness within Bhutan's legal code of 1729, and the articulation of GNH by the Fourth King in the 1970s, to the modern-day integration of GNH within national surveys and policymaking tools, to the application of GNH within new sectors in Bhutan and abroad, the collective learning and understanding of how to create a society based on happiness and well-being have been steadily growing. The road toward a well-being economy has not been without its ups and downs, and as the country modernizes, new challenges are being faced. Emerging social problems include youth unemployment, rapid rural-urban migration, and the influx of global influences that are now entering the country through the internet and social media.

As one Bhutanese minister put it, Bhutan "cannot be a GNH bubble in a GDP world"—words that ring true whether considering the impacts of global warming on this carbon-negative country, or the growing exposure to consumerist culture facing its youth. To this end, Bhutan's expanding CSO community is playing an important role in ensuring that GNH values and principles are embodied at a grassroots level, which will need to be a vital source of innovation moving into the future. Each of the GNH bodies mentioned above will also have a critical role to play in ensuring that the country's focus on well-being remains strong and adaptive to emerging challenges—while simultaneously contributing to the growing global momentum to advance well-being approaches.

To learn more, go to: *www.gnhcentrebhutan.org; https://vimeo.com/85855298*

Case Study From Nova Scotia, Canada

Measuring What Matters

Based on contributions at the Bellagio convening from
Danny Graham, CEO,
Engage Nova Scotia, Canada

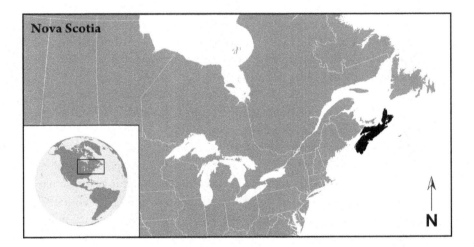

Introduction

For decades, the narrative in Canada's Nova Scotia province has centered on concepts of economic sluggishness and a dwindling population base. This pervasive and unmotivating "we're falling behind" story is built squarely on measures of economic growth, and on the assumption that growing the economy is what matters most. Lost in that formula, however, are qualities that make Nova Scotia a place its residents deeply value. Education levels are high in the province, as are measures for quality of life and community belonging. The region boasts abundant natural beauty. By many counts, Nova Scotia has already achieved the kind of success that other regions would aspire to. And yet, measures that evaluate economic progress ignore this richness.

People in Nova Scotia want to make their province a better place, but many don't feel able to be part of the solutions or know where to begin, especially in this defeatist, economics-dominant context. So leaders in the province launched Engage Nova Scotia, an independent nongovernmental organization (supported by public, private, community, and academic funding) designed to redefine and rediscover what success really means. It is building clarity and confidence behind a new story of what success means and how the province will pursue it, together. Engage Nova Scotia is in its early stages, and yet is already asking questions that are relevant for diverse socio-political contexts.

Context Snapshot

- <u>Leadership:</u> This initiative is NGO-led, in coordination with a coalition of public, private, and NGO partners. It began through investments from the private sector, the Community Foundation of Nova Scotia, and the provincial government, the latter of which nominated one of its staff to serve as the organization's first employee.
- <u>Stage of change:</u> Launched in 2013, Engage Nova Scotia is in the middle stages of defining its measurement approach, informed heavily by grassroots engagement, and in the early stages of applying it as a change strategy. Its household survey in 2019 and resulting reports across 230 data points, expected in 2020, will serve as a foundation for deeper engagement.
- <u>Emphasis:</u> This work is grounded in measurement and focused on narrative change as a key strategy for shifting the way progress is defined and advanced. Its change framework is anchored on three pillars: public engagement, capacity building, and narrative change.

Defining and Measuring Well-Being

The idea of building a new measurement framework was gradually moving from the margins to the mainstream in Nova Scotia 10 years ago but stalled out. Engage Nova Scotia draws on insights from that earlier attempt, adding a very strong commitment to engaging the community to define measures and approaches. When a provincial survey asked, "How should we measure success?" 81 percent of respondents said, "improving our quality of life," whereas 68 percent said, "growing our economy." And yet, measurements of quality of life as an overarching organizing value had been lacking in policy discussions and other decision-making.

Engage Nova Scotia is building a new measurement framework that more fully encompasses the well-being of its people, using a "what, so what, now what?" model. For example, well-being data that aggregate a variety of topics (an example of "what") are imperative for understanding quality of life more broadly. These data may in turn support narrative shifts about what success entails beyond purely economic terms, and build expectations and demand for decisions based on well-being (an example of "so what"). Ultimately, this will lead to pilot projects, broad initiatives, and social changes that enhance well-being (an example of "now what").

Some early actions to create the right data set included disaggregating Canadian Index of Wellbeing (CIW) data and isolating trends for the province since 1994, then releasing that data as the Nova Scotia Quality of Life Index (*www.nsqualityoflife.ca*). It then released "Satisfaction with Life/Happiness" data for each of 55 communities across the province.

Continuous and rigorous new measurement and analysis are priorities for Engage Nova Scotia, as informed by best practices from other jurisdictions. In 2019, Engage Nova Scotia launched a first-of-its-kind household survey, sent to 80,000 residents and designed according to the eight domains and 64 indicators of the CIW. The survey encompasses topics such as loneliness, discrimination, life satisfaction, work-life balance, and healthy work conditions. The survey will expand measures for progress far beyond traditional economic concepts. The high sample size ensures that populations too often under-represented in such research are included, and that data can be disaggregated to identify unique opportunities and challenges within population groups.

Results show that satisfaction with life is higher in Nova Scotia than in Canada as a whole, and higher in rural than urban communities. However, the issue of happiness inequality is greater in Nova Scotia than in all other provinces but one, despite a generally high sense of community belonging, illuminating nuances for further exploration. Engage Nova Scotia aims to continue fine-tuning its ability to call out indicators in its reports where specific demographic groups are performing well below average (analysis and communication that is done in partnership with these groups), underscoring the emphasis on equity.

Engage Nova Scotia is creating tools that "democratize" these data about well-being, making it accessible and meaningful to people across the province. It is working with teams in 10 regions to build capacity for local leaders, including those from communities traditionally excluded from decision-making, to act on the results of the survey before releasing the data widely. Results will be shared in 10 reports in 2020, each of which will support innovative priority setting for the region for years to come. Engage Nova Scotia and its partners will use the data and these reports to prioritize pilot projects that benefit people in each of the province's 10 regions.

Cultural Narrative

Nova Scotians have a reputation for being friendly, tolerant, and plain-spoken. It is often said that they are less focused on material success than other regions of North America. And while partisanship persists, the political discourse is not as polarized as elsewhere on the continent. These conditions foster an enabling cultural environment that may facilitate the initiative's success.

While this work is not yet sufficiently challenging the status quo to have experienced strong resistance, there has been early skepticism from some decision-makers and members of the public alike. Sample comments include: "This is too esoteric. The 'Average Joe' won't see this as relevant." "If you grow jobs, you'll grow happiness." "This is too left-leaning for the mainstream." "I can't see concrete actions flowing from measurements." "Aggregate data sets are inherently flawed." More work is needed to acknowledge and moderate this skepticism, and to advance a narrative that will help to embolden collective success.

Two forces are propelling narrative shift: First, the growing global, national, and local discourse about the unintended by-products of market-driven economies. And second, emerging research about the importance of improving social capital—enhancing community vitality, social integration, a sense of belonging, social trust, and strong relationships.

Grassroots Engagement and Shifting Power
to Build Equity

Committed to being in continual dialogue with the public, Engage Nova Scotia wanted to ensure that its measurement efforts and data releases sparked conversation, inquiry, and action. It followed the release of the Nova Scotia Quality of Life Index with comprehensive public engagement, stakeholder consultation, and communication that encompasses news media, social media, and grassroots outreach. The tone is empowering and inquisitive rather than "educating" or "declaring truths." Each engagement begins by asking questions, then follows people's own perspectives and priorities to surface topics for discussion. This interplay helps fine tune well-being definitions and measurements, illuminate priorities for action, and, most importantly, ensure that the effort belongs to and is shaped by Nova Scotians.

In addition to broad grassroots engagement, collaboration with specific populations with unique needs, strengths, and priorities ensures that all voices are heard and that measurement and actions are tailored to unique cultural contexts. For example, recognizing that Indigenous communities, African Nova Scotians, youth, and people with differing abilities (among other communities) are too often under-represented in surveys, Engage Nova Scotia has consulted with representatives of each group to mobilize representation from their communities in the 2019 survey. Later, together, they will analyze the data, design pilot projects, and set priorities together with those groups.

Partners are also encouraged to experiment and try pilot projects they design, according to criteria of readiness, impact, and the likelihood that results will offer cogent learnings. By sharing success stories and lessons learned along the way, partners will be learning from each other and adapting in order to enhance their effectiveness over time.

Collaboration Among Government, Civil Service, and Research

Engage Nova Scotia is building a coalition from diverse sectors. The coalition is supported by an advisory group that represents the fields of environmental conservation, poverty alleviation, and social services, and that spans disciplines such as academia (including the province's largest university), business alliances and chambers of commerce, nonprofits, county and city governments, public-private partnerships, and many more. The Nova Scotian government is a supporter and partial funder for the work, but is not its leader. This reduces the risk that the initiative will be politicized or vulnerable to shifting priorities through leadership transitions or other "political hijacking," and gives the coalition's partners the freedom to lead and to remain nimble.

Results

An important early milestone is the diverse coalition of partners who have signed on to participate and help lead this endeavor. In addition, social service agencies have already begun to incorporate resulting data into their strategic planning.

The provincial government has begun articulating the need for "inclusive economic growth," a phrase associated with tackling inequity, and an important shift in the direction of broader success measures.

Coalition partners furthermore speak about the agenda and goals of this work in myriad settings, which is already advancing a unified and reinforcing message about the importance of this work and this broader definition of progress.

Instructive Insights for Others Pursuing a Well-Being Approach

Engage Nova Scotia has clarified three principles that are core to the coalition's early success. First, they are firmly focused on the long term, on "going slow to go long." The nature of this work requires a deep and integrated "root structure" of partners who will take on and sustain this work for decades, not try to create short-term actions and declare victory. Engage Nova Scotia is thus cultivating a diverse coalition of influential players, while building trust with potential critics. Partners likewise take authentic approaches when engaging communities on these topics, beginning conversations with questions rather than pronouncements.

Second, the coalition recognizes the overarching arc required for success and where they are on that arc at a given point in time. As they move from measurement to narrative change to advancing specific initiatives, they are growing the field of partners that they need to be successful along the way. They realize that if they were to try to do too much too early, without appreciating the iterative nature of the work, progress could too easily stall.

Third, and in keeping with their value for data-driven solutions, partners are focused on prototyping concrete projects in priority areas that may serve as visible "proofs of concept" to make this work tangible and irrefutable. Storytelling about these projects has the added benefit of reinforcing messages about the agenda and goal at every opportunity.

The Road Ahead

As Nova Scotia continues to assess well-being and apply insights to inform action, it is starting to create tools that "democratize" the data. For example, it will release an online tool related to the survey results, and is working with teams in each of 10 regions in advance of this release to build capacity for local leaders to act on the results of the survey.

As a course correction to the limits of market-driven priority setting, the province's well-being approach is showing strong promise. Engage Nova Scotia continues to build out and advance the strategies in this case study, remaining open to continual learning and adaptation of narrative, strategies, civic engagement, and partner collaboration.

To learn more, go to: *www.engagenovascotia.ca*

Case Study From Palestine

Well-Being in the Context of Chronic Conflict

Based on contributions at the Bellagio convening from
Rita Giacaman, Professor,
Institute of Community and Public Health, Birzeit University, Palestine

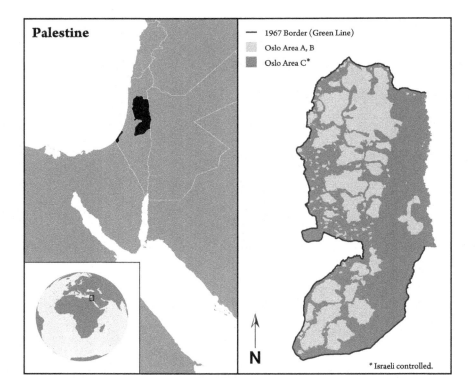

Introduction

Conflict and trauma are constant features of the socio-political landscape in the Palestinian Territories. From a very young age, people across society witness and experience various levels of violence and insecurity on a daily basis. Simple acts, such as going to school or work, can result in movement restrictions, arrest, or detention. While each person internalizes these painful experiences in individual ways, Palestinians also suffer from a communal trauma.

Navigating this emotional terrain requires a collective effort. Palestinian people are often raised in tightly knit extended families and communities that influence their identity. Survival mechanisms and the concepts of rights and responsibilities take shape at collective levels. It follows, then, that collective exposure to trauma affects culture, expectations, and well-being.

Faced with this difficult political context, Palestinian civil society is leading the response to this communal trauma in times of crises, and those are frequent.

The Institute of Community and Public Health based in Birzeit, north of Jerusalem, has been central to this effort in working to understand what happens to people in wars and conflicts. The Institute's work starts by recognizing that Palestinian well-being must be addressed as a communal project. The Institute has found that the biomedical, mental disease-based model for "treating" trauma at individual levels has not proved helpful. Instead, the Institute helps people and groups understand their trauma in collective, socio-political terms. This begins with identifying the political determinants of health as part of the social determinants of health; these conditions interact with biological predisposition to produce disease. From this knowledge base, the Institute uses partnerships and adaptive approaches to establish and spin off pilot projects designed to address societal trauma and improve Palestinians' well-being in ways tailored to their reality. This is a vivid example of the concept that well-being approaches—and well-being itself—look very different in different contexts.

Context Snapshot

- Leadership: Absent operational and sustainable national policy action, the work described here is led by civil society, including at Birzeit University's Institute of Community and Public Health working with the Community Based Rehabilitation consortia of local NGOs.
- Stage of change: The Institute and its partners have worked on interventions and practices to address mental health and well-being since the late 1990s. Its work on new measures of suffering is in the beginning stages.
- Emphasis: This work is focused on research-based understandings of what happens to people in wars and conflicts and community interventions.

Defining and Measuring Well-Being

The Institute of Community and Public Health conceives of well-being and "ill-being" as stages on a continuum on which people oscillate back and forth as conditions change—whether changes in violence and insecurity, or positive changes, like enhanced community connectedness, access to warm and loving relationships, or having people to talk with about problems. (The notion of "ill-being" includes the "internal or invisible wounds" that result from repeated and chronic exposure to political violence; these invisible wounds threaten well-being and can even lead to disease over the course of one's lifetime.) Standard well-being measures fall short under these circumstances, so the Institute and its partners have developed culturally and contextually relevant indicators and metrics to evaluate conditions of suffering, such as distress and insecurity, and to explore how each affects people's subjective well-being. Well-being data are then compiled by engaging people through personal interviews and focus groups to collect quantitative data, and the Institute provides the training and support that make it possible. Sample questions include:

On "individual distress":
- To what extent do you feel unable to control the important things in your life?
- To what extent did you feel humiliated?
- To what extent do you feel fed up with life?

On "human insecurity":
- To what extent do you fear for yourself in your daily life?
- To what extent do you worry/fear about losing your home?
- To what extent does your family feel fear for your safety?

The Institute's research shows that its locally-developed measures are more effective at assessing quality of life in Palestine than global measures, i.e., the World Health Organization (WHO) Quality of Life Brief. Whereas WHO's measure could not detect changes among the Gaza population, human insecurity and distress significantly increased from 2005 to 2009, as illuminated by the Institute's research.

Cultural Narrative

In Palestine, narratives around well-being are about *context* over culture—specifically, a context defined by enduring warlike conditions experienced by the Palestinian people. The Institute works to change the narrative around social suffering from one that pathologizes it as a matter of individual mental health (something that happens "between your ears") and instead as a consequence of acute, sustained, and collectively experienced conflict. This context of conflict profoundly influences people's well-being, not merely their state of mind.

While context shapes Palestinians' well-being, culture—and a sense of history—is also a factor that influences how people understand trauma. Palestinians have endured and resisted their conditions for decades. In many ways, people have become normalized to their conditions in order to study, work, create families, and survive. The challenge with this survival mechanism is that it can diminish one's sense of agency. This dichotomy creates an opportunity to continue harnessing Palestinians' perspective in order to further build capacity to endure and resist conditions that counter well-being. (At the Institute, "endure and resist" is preferred to "resilience," which implies going back to where you began.)

Grassroots Engagement and Shifting Power to Build Equity

In a context lacking strong national policy action, and where political priorities too often respond to emergencies and/or funder priorities (both of which may shift dramatically from year to year), resulting policies are rarely feasible, operational, or sustainable. The Institute's work is therefore designed to create change from the ground up, working in partnership with local and international NGOs that have deep grassroots reach. Their model respects communities' agency for improving conditions and building power at the local level; the Institute and its partners see themselves as facilitating changes that communities create for themselves.

The Institute and its partners undertake a range of community-based activities beginning with needs assessments that test, adapt, and apply international measures and create new measures relevant to local context and culture where needed. They train community workers in areas such as how to conduct needs assessments in order to develop interventions, which require some training in qualitative and sometimes quantitative methods; how to set up records generated from interventions and how to assess them and use them for future planning; and practical skills, such as psychosocial group counseling. They also provide ongoing mentorship and supervision, among other activities. Their experience shows that when pilot programs are successful, others will model and scale up those approaches, spurring practice changes even without policy changes that would promote it.

Collaboration Among Government, Civil Service, and Research

The Institute's role in local partnerships is frequently to put research at the core of well-being interventions. Its partners include the Community Based Rehabilitation (CBR) program of the Palestinian Medical Relief Society, the Health Work Committees, the Palestinian Counseling Center, Patients' Friends Society, and the Red Crescent Society. The Institute supports these organizations, among others, through research, training, and supervision.

The health and well-being of adolescent Palestinians is one priority area for the Institute's partnerships, in part because young people have been at the forefront of daily conflict. By 2002, the Institute began conducting research on aggregate shifts in mental health among 15- to 29-year-olds. During the Second Palestinian Uprising (2000–2004), the team observed a rise in mental health problems among this group. To address this, in cooperation with CBR and others, the Institute introduced youth groups facilitated by CBR workers and designed to alleviate stressors and mental health problems that surfaced in their research. It is during these discussions that an important epiphany often occurs: The symptoms or negative feelings one holds are shared by others; their experience is not a personal one, but rather socio-political. Additional interventions include practice changes (such as the integration of psychosocial health into horizontal programs), and developing support systems that allow participants to learn from each other and overcome problems together—thereby reducing social isolation and stigma while promoting stress relief.

Throughout these partnerships, the work is guided by a principle of listening to and learning from people, and leveraging the trusted relationships that community members and local NGOs have built through decades of community service and support.

Results

Some of these partnerships have inspired new interventions at scale. For example, collaboration between the Institute and local NGOs in the late 1980s helped to establish women's health programs that continue today. These programs were successful in part because they used research and evaluation as an integral part of the strategy, driving adaptations in real time. In part because of these programs—along with the parallel efforts of an NGO-driven women's movement that called for change by marrying model programs with advocacy—the Palestinian Ministry of Health established a women's health directorate and program. Many local NGOs did the same.

Those engaged in the Institute's work increasingly see value in well-being measures and data collection to inform interventions and practices. There is also increased agency and voice from community members in program design. Given the central role that civil service and research play in improving conditions for Palestinian people, positive shifts in these realms hold promise for continued progress in the pursuit of well-being in the region.

Instructive Insights for Others Pursuing a Well-Being Approach

Definitions and measurements of well-being differ dramatically according to cultural, social, and political context. To promote well-being effectively, interventions must deeply understand—and be informed by the community experiencing—these contexts to ensure that solutions are appropriate, practical, accepted, and successful.

The Road Ahead

The Institute continues its work in close cooperation with partners, such as identifying the various factors associated with well-being and developing locally relevant measures to assess outcomes. In the next five years, they will refine a range of new measures that will link experiences to traumas and outcomes. These include: an experience of racism measure; a "silencing" measure (e.g., stories about how violence affects Palestinians are often ignored by news and academic media and others); and an "uncertainty" measure (e.g., uncertainty whether the way to work will be blocked by a checkpoint, uncertainty around curfews, and individual safety and that of one's family). As they continue to develop locally relevant measures that clarify what happens to people in wars and conflicts, they will publish their results and adapt trainings accordingly.

At the same time, the Institute is intensifying training on issues such as how to expand health strategies from biomedical dichotomies toward a well-being continuum. Training is also expanding around qualitative and quantitative research skills, record-keeping, and needs assessments, among others in response to needs as they arise. The Institute will also continue to publish papers to share research results in order to influence local policies, whenever possible, as well as international aid policies in the country and the Middle East more broadly.

To learn more, go to: *http://icph.birzeit.edu*

Case Study From Singapore

Inspiring the Next Generation of Leaders to Prioritize Well-Being

Based on contributions at the Bellagio convening from
Kee-Seng Chia, Founding Dean and Professor,
Saw Swee Hock School of Public Health, National University of Singapore

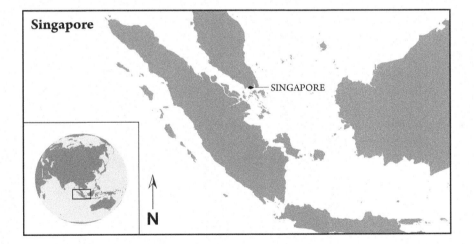

Introduction

In the decades since Singapore's independence in 1965, the nation has transformed from one facing basic challenges related to sanitation and disease prevention, to a world-class economy and a gold standard for health care. Factors that contribute to this trajectory include a stable government with a long-term vision of how Singapore should grow economically, guided by a high-level Economic Review Panel of global and local business leaders, international and local academics, and political officeholders. This group meets periodically to chart the direction of Singapore's economic growth by projecting two to three decades into the future.

While this approach has brought tremendous gains for the country and its people, an unintended consequence of this economics-first approach has been the reinforcement of values and narratives that equate financial *wealth* with *success*. And while health has improved across a range of indicators in the process, it nevertheless remains a distant second as a values driver in both national decision-making and in the choices Singaporeans make daily. In many instances, young working adults often pursue wealth at the expense of their health, not recognizing that their current unhealthy lifestyle will result in chronic diseases as they age.

Leaders in the School of Public Health at the National University of Singapore recognized the urgent need to shift the value system among the next generation of leaders. If health became a value at least equal to wealth, they reasoned, this shift would pave the way for a different expectation, demand, set of behaviors, and, ultimately, policies that advance well-being. These efforts are beginning through a partnership called the "Healthy Campus Initiative" (HCI), which is designed to serve as a pilot project for broader community-focused efforts. HCI is currently being developed in the two major universities in Singapore—the National University of Singapore and the Nanyang Technological University—in collaboration with the Ministry of Health Office of Healthcare Transformation.

HCI's vision: to raise cohorts of university graduates by 2025 who embrace a value system that gives equal emphasis to health and wealth, and who will serve as lifelong ambassadors for promoting well-being in society. This new generation of workplace and community leaders will inspire a social movement toward healthy lifestyles as a default by shaping policies and programs that advance well-being. Ultimately the initiative will accelerate broader approaches for stemming the epidemic of chronic disease in the country and advance societal well-being.

Context Snapshot

- <u>Leadership:</u> The Healthy Campus Initiative is led by two universities in close collaboration with the Ministry of Health Office of Healthcare Transformation. Within each university, leadership is provided by administrative enterprises reporting to the presidents. The universities aim to draw in other components of the academic enterprise to support and evaluate programs.
- <u>Stage of change:</u> This work is in nascent stages.
- <u>Emphasis:</u> This work is focused on shifting narratives and mindsets among future leaders.

Defining and Measuring Well-Being

Because of the wealth-first mentality, economic measures dominate in Singapore; well-being is not currently defined or measured at the national level.

Specific to HCI, objectives are necessarily long-term; it is explicitly *not* intended to achieve immediate performance indicators. Measures track progress toward longer-term cultural and narrative shifts, including:

- Establishing an HCI office on each campus to drive co-creation and delivery of solutions at the campus level.
- Developing a "health examination system" for incoming and graduating students to measure the extent to which students lead healthier lives as they leave the university than they did when they entered.
- Promoting academic research to measure shifts in societal values and priorities around health.

Cultural Narrative

At the national level, the political narrative has expanded beyond wealth to a more inclusive definition of success. This is accelerated by the transformation to a "Smart Nation" and efforts to better use technology to improve ideas, applications, and solutions. Achieving this goal requires a population that is resilient in both health and wealth, and national policies that achieve both economic growth and population well-being.

At its heart, HCI is a narrative change initiative. The idea is that by changing the narrative among future leaders about what matters and how people define, measure, and pursue success, this effort will propel a lasting shift in values, mindsets, and behaviors—both individual and societal.

Changing the narrative, of course, requires far more than a new story or set of messages. HCI uses a three-pronged strategy to shift students' experiences and perceptions, creating a different reality that over time becomes the accepted narrative about what matters. The three strategies are: (1) fostering a whole-of-campus culture among students and staff that values healthy living; (2) creating an environment that makes healthy living the default on these campuses; and (3) catalyzing a supportive operating system that elevates health in decision-making, from campus policies to management.

Changing the culture among university students is challenging because their views have already been shaped by broader cultural norms and values. For example, it is ingrained in young people that success in life begins with a university degree; consequently, for the 25 percent of young people who successfully gain university entrance, academic excellence often ranks above all else.

Some argue that efforts to inculcate this new culture and value system should begin even earlier, among primary and secondary school children. HCI affirms, however, that undergraduates and recent graduates are at a pivotal stage of transition, so remain an important focus for cultural narrative work. As students move out of the direct influence of their parents and grandparents—people who frequently contributed to Singapore's success, and may espouse values for wealth at the expense of health—those students are increasingly questioning their culture's values and are open to finding their own goals and direction in life. Universities and workplaces therefore remain strategic avenues for shaping the value systems of young adults—who will go on to raise the next generation.

Grassroots Engagement and Shifting Power to Build Equity

A key principle in developing scalable and sustainable policies and programs is community engagement and ownership. Historically, when Singapore was under-developed and lacked natural resources, there was a strong dependence on top-down directions and decisions to drive the country forward. In the last two decades, however, with a more educated and empowered population, there has been greater involvement and dialogue between the government and the people it governs.

For example, the "Singapore Conversation," a 2012 national initiative, involved more than 47,000 Singaporeans who participated in more than 660 dialogues island-wide. The purpose of those discussions was to identify Singaporeans' priorities, values, concerns, and preferences. New legislation, like enhanced tobacco control measures, went through numerous rounds of public consultations prior to their presentation to the legislature.

The HCI will similarly conduct workshops and classes to sensitize students and staff to key concepts and to solicit their ideas and ownership. Such engagement will require time, and must occur early in the initiative.

Collaboration Among Government and Research

The opportunity for greater collaboration between academia and government in public health policies and programs arose in 2011 when the Ministry of

Health supported the formation of a national School of Public Health at the National University of Singapore. The school initially contributed to two major policies: the War on Diabetes and Total Workplace Safety and Health.

The War on Diabetes used Type II Diabetes as the focal point for non-communicable disease control in Singapore. A major strategy is on primary prevention—promoting increased physical activity and healthy diets at the national level. This required a whole-of-government as well as a whole-of-society approach, tackling the problem at societal, communal, and household levels.

In parallel, the Total Workplace Safety and Health initiative brings the problem of chronic disease prevention and management to employers and workers. It integrates safety, occupational diseases, general health issues, and well-being of workers under a single management and framework.

These two initiatives surfaced the need to develop a new generation of employers and business leaders who value health and well-being just as much as wealth; the HCI is one of the first steps in this direction. HCI fits into the Ministry of Health Office of Healthcare Transformation's aim to test scalable initiatives to achieve health systems reform, which it articulates as the "three beyonds." That is: beyond hospitals and into communities (shifting the focus of health care away from hospitals to community care); beyond "quality" and toward "value" (ensuring effective care while mitigating spiraling health care costs); and beyond health care to health (emphasis on primary prevention and promotion of health and well-being).

Instructive Insights for Others Pursuing a Well-Being Approach

In Singapore, as in other settings, there is an emphasis on efforts with visible activities, actions, and results, and this emphasis can be distracting for longer-term efforts. To be successful there is a need to engage various stakeholders with a common long-term vision, especially the students and staff who are recipients of the programs and policies.

There is also a need to work with the universities' academic side since HCI offers opportunities for teaching and research, particularly translational research to create new therapies, medical procedures, or diagnostics. Here, as in other settings, there is some perception among academic staff that translational research is less valued than basic research. The National University of Singapore has therefore started an HCI Translation Research Unit to engage academic staff who have a passion for translation and who are not under the pressure of seeking tenure to spearhead research projects that will help HCI achieve its mission.

The Road Ahead

Collaborators remain focused on the vision of new generations of leaders who value health and well-being. Along the way, the Office of Healthcare Transformation hopes specific HCI frameworks, tools, and programs may be scaled and adopted at wider community and national levels. Additionally, challenges related to implementation invite a new academic discipline: that of implementation science.

For more information, contact: Professor Kee-Seng Chia (*ephcks@nus.edu.sg*).

Case Study From the United Kingdom

Making What Matters Count

Based on contributions at the Bellagio convening from
Liz Zeidler, Chief Executive,
Happy City,* United Kingdom

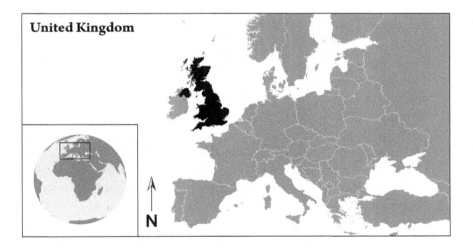

Introduction

For most people, well-being is understood and experienced at a local scale. Their community or city is where housing, green spaces, social cohesion, mental health, and many other vital elements of well-being play out in daily life. Local governments and other stakeholders also tend to be the most willing and able to try innovative approaches. Local wins, in turn, inform and inspire action in other areas and often build to national change.

---

* Happy City's work focuses on England and Wales, but its survey is used across the United Kingdom.

Recognizing the potential power of local action to spur a well-being economy, in 2010, visionary thinkers in the United Kingdom established Happy City, a nonprofit organization with a lofty goal: "To make what matters count."

This approach is based on the premise that "if we measure the wrong things, we strive for the wrong things."* Money and economic growth are means, not ends, and they must be used as enablers, not drivers, of our society. Happy City works with city and municipal governments and other key place-based stakeholders to put "thriving lives" as the central goal at the heart of decision-making.

No one size fits all. Since the Second World War, migration to the United Kingdom has resulted in ever-more diverse populations. In Bristol alone, where Happy City is based, 91 different languages are spoken in the schools. Happy City therefore puts a significant emphasis on grassroots engagement across all cultures to define what really matters to people, customize a measurement framework, and apply insights to improve well-being.

Context Snapshot

- <u>Leadership:</u> Happy City is a U.K.-based charity working with local and municipal governments to provide measurement, training, and consulting. Local-level leadership looks different in the context of each place but is largely government-led with significant involvement of civil society.
- <u>Stage of change:</u> Started in Bristol in 2010, Happy City now offers assessments for 373 local authorities across the United Kingdom.
- <u>Emphasis:</u> Happy City begins with measurement, defining and using new measures to "shift the compass" to well-being. Increasingly it is also helping municipalities and others apply the data to create place-based change.

Defining and Measuring Well-Being

Happy City offers two main well-being measurement tools: the Thriving Places Index and the Happiness Pulse survey.

The Thriving Places Index provides a framework for evaluating and reporting the conditions for well-being at local levels, including:

- Local conditions, which encompass a diverse array of indicators, such as place and environment (e.g., green space, safety, housing), mental and physical

---

* Joseph Stiglitz Report by the Commission on the Measurement of Economic Performance and Social Progress 2008.

health, education and learning, work and local economy, and people and community (e.g., social networks, civic engagement, and community cohesion).
- Equality, e.g., health inequality, income inequality, social mobility.
- Sustainability, e.g., CO_2 emissions, household recycling, and energy consumption.

Sample measures include:

- *Good jobs:* Not just employment/unemployment levels, but also the percentage of employment that provides secure jobs, a living wage, and neither under- nor overworked hours.
- *Community cohesion:* Levels of "social fragmentation" measured via the percentage of people who move to a new house each year or who live alone.
- *Social mobility:* Measure academic achievement and quality of nurseries and schools for those in the lower percentile of economic status.

To complement the Index data (which focuses on the conditions for well-being), Happy City also provides the Happiness Pulse to gather subjective data on people's experienced lives. This five-minute, online survey of community residents explores how people think and feel about their lives, what they do that supports better lives, and how they connect with others. Sample survey questions and statements:

- *Be:* "I've been feeling optimistic about the future lately." "I've been feeling useful." "I've been dealing with problems well."
- *Do:* "How often do you spend 30 minutes playing sports or physical exercise?" "How often do you spend time informally learning about something new?" "I notice and appreciate the little things in life."
- *Connect:* "How often do you meet socially with friends, relatives, or work colleagues?" "How often do you feel lonely?" "Do you have friend/s or family member/s with whom you can discuss personal matters?" "I feel like I belong to this neighborhood."

The Pulse tool is used by organizations large and small as well as municipalities to map well-being strengths and needs, and to evaluate the impact of projects on the lives of those in their community. Happy City supports local leaders and organizations to understand and apply the data to inform action.

Cultural Narrative

Happy City is designed to challenge head-on the dominant narrative that happiness—and societal progress—is achieved through increased consumption and production. Shifting the narrative about what matters, and what can provide happiness and contentment, can disrupt the relentless drive for consumption.

Through its national communication work and local training and consulting, Happy City is working to put a new goal—supporting thriving people on a thriving planet—as the "north star" for policy and action. By making this shift in cultural narrative and in decision-making, it aims to create a ripple effect that will influence all aspects of people's lives, from education to cities designed for social cohesion.

Grassroots Engagement and Shifting Power to Build Equity

A commitment to equity is at the core of this work. Happy City makes its tools accessible to all (in terms of content, presentation style, and reach) and ensures that its outreach engages perspectives across the community. By design, the Thriving Places Index can never be reduced to a single "well-being" score, as doing so would too easily conceal inequalities or unsustainable approaches.

Along the way, Happy City is guided by two grassroots principles. First, start with people. Happy City began by engaging a diverse cross-section of the U.K. population, visiting gatherings and locations including prisons, refugee groups, parents' groups, shopping centers, and businesses. It embarked on this listening tour to understand what really matters to people, how they viewed and found well-being in their lives, and to envision together what a thriving place would look like. From this public consultation, Happy City worked with leading academics and policymakers to define measures of what matters to people. This gave the program a solid ground for designing solutions, and an authentic story to underpin its practical measurement tools.

Second, Happy City designs trainings, communication, and measurement tools that work for everyone. All of its work must pass a critical litmus test: "Would this work as well for the most under-served person as well as it would for the mayor?"

Collaboration Among Government, Civil Service, and Research

The success of this approach is contingent on building alliances. Happy City has gathered people from diverse sectors who share a commitment to a well-being approach, new economics, place-making, and other means of improving the world where they live. Its partners include academics, policymakers, thought leaders, and, crucially, frontline workers who test, shape, challenge, and inform everything it does.

Key players include:

- Local governments, particularly those working with a cross-sector, place-based approach and that are open to innovation. Happy City has found that bold and open leadership at both political and managerial levels is vital to creating the conditions for radical new ways of defining progress to take root.
- Civil society organizations, including those working on the ground to deliver local projects to enhance well-being, as well as "umbrella" groups that support and fund local work. When these influencers embrace a well-being approach, it is often eye-opening for others.
- Funders and commissioners, including those who donate to Happy City, such as the National Lottery Community Fund.
- Public and civil society organizations that commission research and consultancy, such as Public Health England and the Office for National Statistics. Their influence helps move new approaches from the margins and into policy and practice.
- Businesses, particularly those that already recognize their role in society beyond private profit margins, and that are willing to work with other sectors to support local action. Such businesses lend credibility to the use of a well-being framework.
- Academics and think tanks, including consortia such as the What Works Centre for Wellbeing and the U.K.-based, international Centre for the Understanding of Sustainable Prosperity. These institutions offer evidence that validates new measures and that often gives decision-makers the confidence to make decisions in the collective interest.

Results

Happy City publishes the Thriving Places Index results for 373 local authorities in England and Wales each year, and is working with 12 of those local authorities areas to fully embed this framework into their operations. More and more places are using this integrated cycle of measurement, understanding, and adaptation, building a strong set of learnings and case studies.

One example of how shifting the measurement compass is influencing policy and program action is in Birmingham, the second-largest city in the United Kingdom. As the city, led by the Active Wellbeing Society, embarked on a three-year program to support some of the most disadvantaged communities to get more physically active, it started working with Happy City and using the Thriving Places Index to understand how actions to increase physical activity also affect other aspects of life such as education, social cohesion, people's relationship to nature and to sustainability, and their relationship to health and to the economy. With this information, the city is better able to design policies and programs with broad impact—and to measure that impact holistically.

At the individual level, more than 30,000 people have taken the Happiness Pulse survey so far, representing participation across regional, organizational, public, private, and civil society perspectives, and from groups both large and small. Happy City has now adapted the technology to allow it to be scaled at pace across the whole of the United Kingdom, and beyond.

Instructive Insights for Others Pursuing a Well-Being Approach

This work has surfaced a few challenges that merit proactive effort to address. For example, political priorities at national and local levels are ever-changing, and follow political "fashion cycles" that seem to shorten with time. Policymakers can get caught up in individual issues that are vital but that represent singular aspects of well-being (e.g., loneliness, cohesion, obesity, air quality, and more); leveraging that interest while staying true to the holistic intention of this work is a fine balancing act.

Along the way, Happy City works to balance the need for local adaptation and co-creation with the risk of well-being measurement becoming too complex and variable. Providing rigorous yet practical core tools, while staying highly adaptable and easily understandable, increases the potential for taking the approach to scale and mobilizing more substantive societal change.

Happy City also engages the "person behind the role," leaning into the values and humanity of decision-makers. For example, most people would say their ultimate desire for their children is for them to be happy. Many leaders would say that the end goal of a good society is to help people thrive. This work aims to tap into this universal wisdom, and to help people see beyond the economic and political constructs that too often cloak their pursuit of progress.

An additional challenge is insufficient funding for "radical" ideas. This work is, by design, challenging the systems that enable and perpetuate wealth for so many mainstream sources of philanthropy. Funders have been reluctant to support work that, when successful, may undermine systems driving their own wealth. There are, however, reasons to be hopeful that this is changing.

The Road Ahead

Happy City's focus is on supporting shifts among the major levers of change needed to transform organizations and places nationwide. It provides guidance on well-being budgeting and leadership training in well-being economics, and supports the integration of other models (such as Sustainable Development Goals) into a well-being economy approach.

The organization has adapted its tools to deliver at scale across the United Kingdom. The online Pulse tool now has the capacity for any organization, large or small, to have a unique survey URL and results dashboard, providing the capacity to map well-being strengths and needs and to measure well-being impacts of interventions for thousands of organizations. Custom-built additional Pulse modules can uncover sector-specific impacts for community groups, housing organizations, sport and fitness initiatives, and workplaces. These adaptations (with more in the pipeline) support the ambition for a whole-place approach, enabling all sectors and all sizes of organizations within them to shift to a well-being economy approach.

In response to inquiries from places around the world that want to learn from, adapt, and apply its work, Happy City is expanding its capacity to facilitate application of its models globally. While the cultural and data context varies significantly around the world, the key drivers of well-being remain largely consistent. The core research and accessible framework behind the Happy City tools allow different places to adapt them to fit local needs and data availability. Happy City's team of experts partner with others to share their learning (and that of other cities using the tools), and to promote quality outcomes in new and emerging settings.

At the same time, Happy City continues to play a part in supporting a broader narrative around progress that encompasses well-being, bolstering a growing global movement for change.

To learn more, go to: *www.happycity.org.uk*

REFLECTIONS

Applying and Measuring the Well-Being Framework in the United States

The dynamic conversations and presentations during the week at Bellagio provided the content of this book. The previous chapters conclude that shifting power and building authentic and inclusive opportunities so all people can define and pursue well-being is critically important. Aligning governments, civil society organizations, research, and measurement approaches to prioritize what matters most, as defined by people living in the community, is also essential.

To focus more specifically on how these ideas might play out in the United States, two commentators share their reflections here, bringing both a research perspective and an on-the-ground application, echoing the commitment at Bellagio to learn from both the academy and the field. Laura Kubzansky, professor at the Harvard T.H. Chan School of Public Health, describes the opportunity presented by the asset-based well-being framework for public health, and calls for continued development of the science behind—and the evidence for—well-being approaches. Julia Rusk, former chief of Civic Wellbeing for the city of Santa Monica, California, uses the story of the work happening in her community to reinforce many of the insights in this book, from community-informed measurement and shifts in narrative, to changes in practice and policy.

Afterword

A Vision for Well-Being Policies and Action in the United States, Based on Santa Monica's Experience

JULIA E. RUSK

Former Chief of Civic Wellbeing, City Manager's Office, City of Santa Monica, California

> *We've been wrong about what our job is in medicine. We think our job is to ensure health and survival . . . but really it is to enable well-being. And well-being is about the reasons one wishes to be alive.*
>
> —*Atul Gawande*
> *Being Mortal*

The year is 2030.

In the city of Santa Monica, California, a quick pulse point from social media sources finds that social isolation rates are rising among seniors in assisted living. The data also reveal—almost as a non sequitur—that these seniors miss eating their favorite foods. At the same time, data from Santa Monica's high school show that students whose parents are not college-educated have much higher rates of success when another adult is involved in their lives.[1,2]

Immediately, the city identifies a point person to initiate a "pop-up" program connecting these students with isolated seniors, providing both groups with simple training and support. Within 12 months, the majority of seniors in the group report feeling much less isolated, and the percentage of their student counterparts who go on to college rises by double digits. As an additional bonus, students have gone to the local farmers' market to buy some of the seniors' favorite foods, which they cook together, breaking bread, sharing culture, and improving nutrition and satisfaction in both groups.

This is the future of well-being—one example of how the power of data can illuminate needs and inspire action. Without well-being data, government is working in the dark, unable to swiftly and accurately understand the desires and hopes of the community and improve the quality of life. As of this writing, government almost never addresses how people feel, what their aspirations are, and if an action will improve, worsen, or have no effect on the quality of their daily lives. In short, Gawande's prescription for medicine applies equally to government: The job of government is not merely to ensure the rule of law, catalyze the economy, and fill the proverbial potholes; it is to enable well-being.

But this is not just about data; it is how data can connect the dots, reveal the priorities of community, and kindle solutions. As many authors in this book have highlighted, the purpose of data is to put it into action. Our goal in Santa Monica is to make this a reality, with benefits accruing regularly to every resident, neighborhood, business, and contributor to the community. As interest in well-being approaches gains steam within local governments, our experience—and the others in this book—can offer a path forward, especially for small and mid-size cities like ours.

We know that applying well-being data won't fix everything. But it does provide a robust method for government, especially local government, to rapidly spot issues, implement solutions, and just as rapidly, gauge just how effective those solutions are. The need for strong analysis and innovative problem-solving—that is, caring people paying close attention—remains eternal. Well-being measurements give government a powerful tool to filter the oceans of data, or to collect additional information about how people are doing—not to sell more widgets or to spy on their residents, but for the common good. Well-being measurement can focus the conversation of government on the aspirations and needs of its people, forging hopeful and thoughtful solutions. These new measures help drive a narrative that is more honest about long-standing conditions, biases, and policies that have impeded the ability of many to thrive and flourish, and that point to a different future marked by equity and opportunity.

This was the idea behind Santa Monica's local well-being index: harnessing the power of data for the commonwealth that would reveal the story of the people and the community in new ways, and that would help to transform city government.

What spurred all this? Two profoundly sorrowful incidents.

In November 2009, a 19-year-old who had just finished an evening art class was mistaken for a gang member and shot to death. We began—once again in our community—to address youth violence. Fourteen months later, a ninth grader jumped to his death. These tragedies touched many across our community. We in local government knew we had to expand our reach. We needed to examine not selective sectors, but collective impact. We quickly grasped that we had to understand what was happening with kids and families in the developmental life cycle—from cradle to career. We decided to generate a Report Card on Youth that would help us craft better policy solutions and address these issues with a significantly sharper understanding.

That would require good data.

We began having discussions with young people, parents, educators, police, and health care leaders. We discovered that there already was an enormous amount of data, but it was segmented and sequestered. Educators had data about how many students were graduating; police on who was being arrested; health care systems on who was getting sick; and governments were looking at usage of programs. The easiest thing to do with all this data was drown in it. But nowhere was it all being put together for a community-wide portrait of *overall well-being—a portrait that could be used to forge solutions to our most pressing problems.*

As these conversations and realizations culminated in the summer of 2012, Bloomberg Philanthropies issued its first Mayors Challenge. It was a call for big, bold ideas—innovative proposals in local government with a shot at moving the needle on things that matter—the equivalent of a government X-Prize.

The timing could not have been better.

As work on the Youth Report Card progressed, we thought: Wait, this has broad community impact, not just on kids and their families. What if we scaled what we are doing for youth to work on well-being for the *entire* population?

Research quickly revealed there was related work going on around the world, particularly at a national level—perhaps most famously in Bhutan, but also in the United Kingdom and Canada. But much of the work, we found, was done by research and advocacy groups outside of government.

In 2012, I led the team that began work on a proposal to create the first multidimensional well-being index designed by and for a city government. Nine months and many hurdles later, Bloomberg Philanthropies awarded Santa Monica with a million-dollar innovation grant to develop that index.

We got right to work by hiring a team from the RAND Corporation, headquartered in Santa Monica, and the New Economics Foundation in London, a small think tank that had already been doing well-being work in the United Kingdom.

We started with one of the more elusive aspects of well-being: what it is. We enlisted guidance from a panel of experts. We engaged with a range of community members, volunteers, and business and civic leaders. We listened closely to what matters most to people. We defined well-being across six broad dimensions: personal outlook, community, place and planet, health, lifelong learning, and economic opportunity.

The goal of the well-being index was to expand the measures of a community far beyond the traditional and economically-focused GDP. We wanted to capture the *human experience* of living in Santa Monica, and to quantify life satisfaction.

It was ambitious. But not crazy. In fact, given the abundance of data in the digital age, it seemed crazy *not* to try.

Data came from a range of sources, including numbers about disease rates, parks, libraries, crime, affordability, education levels, and use of transit services. We analyzed social media data by looking at sentiments of positive and negative emotion, and the intensity of these sentiments. Those data were all publicly available, used often by the private sector to sell us stuff, but rarely mined for the public good. Proprietary limitations and privacy concerns always loomed large. Finally, we conducted an online survey to collect information from residents about personal experiences, including life satisfaction, social connections, housing, and health, among other topics. To ensure that this was not merely a data exercise, we started early in discussing the importance of well-being and shaping the story of why well-being matters. We thought about our ambitions for Santa Monica before even embarking on the measurement and data analysis. We wanted to tie the end use of whatever we did to the hopes of the community. This was our initial well-being narrative shift, a concept that is discussed extensively in this book.

As we were doing all this, we were already getting results from the findings from our Youth Report Card, which by then had become the Youth Wellbeing Report Card. We found higher rates of binge-drinking in teens, higher reports of mental health concerns, and racial disparities in academic achievement already showing up in third grade. Yet one of the biggest revelations lay at the nexus of childhood and education: kindergarten readiness. Our overall population of pre-K kids were not anywhere near the kind of ready that we expected.

Now for a bit of context. Though surrounded by Los Angeles, Santa Monica is a small city of 93,000 residents. With the long-standing investments in early childhood programs, great libraries and parks, before- and after-school programs, and other resources to support kids and families, many believed that most five-year-olds in Santa Monica would be "very ready" to enter kindergarten.

What the data revealed was that most children were *not* very ready. What's more, there was a persistent and consistent number who were very vulnerable.

This showed up in the details—the small things that turn out to have enormous implications. It included tasks like holding pencils, and socioeconomic differences, such as individual access to books. It especially appeared on socializing scales, such as being ready to get along with other kids.

The implications of readiness were formidable. It had predictive value for health, education, and social outcomes. Groups of children vulnerable on any one of the scales used in this instrument are more likely to perform below expectation in all academic areas by the fourth grade.

One key component in the Youth Wellbeing Report Card was the ability to disaggregate and understand differences by gender, race, income levels, and zip codes. It was critical to get beyond a citywide view for more "close-ups."

That, in a nutshell, is the great promise of data read through a wellbeing lens: its potential to highlight gaps that traditional measures miss, and to illuminate opportunities to advance equity.

Indeed, the data revealed differences between neighborhoods—and a complicated mix of factors. For example, we found, among other things, that there were vulnerable kids who came from Santa Monica's most affluent neighborhoods. It reminded us of the danger of clinging too tightly to expectations and assumptions, and just how easy it can be to miss significant factors that contribute to issues, especially when we're looking primarily at economic indicators. And as brain science has confirmed what early childhood advocates have long observed, what happens in the early years matters a lot.

As the impetus of our project was to use data to create better impacts, our response to these findings was multi-pronged, spanning programs and practices as well as policies and resource allocation. To start, we created and launched a kindergarten-readiness campaign. This was a set of tools for parents, caregivers, and educators to foster growth in children in social and emotional development, physical and motor skills, language development, and dual-language learning.

Santa Monica public librarians stepped up in a big way. Public libraries are a treasured community resource and enhanced, freely accessible resources for early literacy and parent support programming. The Early Childhood Task Force, a community advocacy group under the aegis of the city, guided and directed pre-school professionals to embed in their programs discussions with parents and tools for enhancing kinder-readiness. And the school system itself, as a part of the realization that preschool and kindergarten needed a stronger connection, changed its district curriculum director's focus from *K–5* to *Pre-k–5*. Schools knew they needed to pay more attention to what was happening in the younger years. And in addition to families learning how to get children "kindergarten ready," elementary schools needed to shift to become ready for kindergarteners. Now they were.

As this work was underway, we completed the framework, data collection, and analysis for the citywide Wellbeing Index. In Spring 2015, we released the first Wellbeing Index findings for the city of Santa Monica.

Again, the data revealed surprises. We learned that a significantly high number of people lacked strong social connections and a sense of neighborhood cohesion. An unexpectedly high percentage felt they had very little influence on local decision-making, despite the fact that residents vote and volunteer at higher-than-average rates. We also discovered a disturbingly low level of personal well-being in young adults, with one in five saying they felt lonely most or all of the time.

The city began addressing these and other findings with a variety of pilot programs and partnerships. One example is the city's Wellbeing Microgrants, designed to foster resident-developed projects to improve community well-being. These have successfully supported more than a dozen innovative projects in the first year, with double that number planned for the second year. In some cases, these Microgrant projects also helped to direct the city to a larger solution, such as creative approaches to entrepreneurial support for low-income residents. What's more, the Wellbeing Microgrants had the unanticipated but powerful effect of creating grassroots champions of well-being.

A second example is the Pico Wellbeing Project, a neighborhood-based initiative using the cross-disciplinary well-being themes and findings to engage residents and create solutions to issues such as gentrification, resident displacement, and even health.

The main advance is that the framework that we originally created for the Wellbeing Index has been adapted to become the guiding structure for the city's 2019–21 two-year budget and new performance management system. This organization-wide use of the well-being framework organizes city departments and operations around well-being dimensions and outcomes. Going forward, the Wellbeing Index will be the tool used to evaluate whether policies, programs, and other city investments are in fact improving community well-being.

We now call Santa Monica a "Sustainable City of Wellbeing." What we have done in Santa Monica is something that any city, town, or community anywhere in the nation, and probably the world, can also achieve. One of the key goals of Bloomberg Philanthropies Mayor's Challenge is to share and spread bold ideas that work. That is much more than good sense and good science. It is how culture change begins.

Centering focus on well-being in every town and state is the vision and the goal. Defining, measuring, and actively improving well-being makes good sense. A Wellbeing Index is a powerful tool to help government with its primary mission: supporting an equitable and thriving community for all. With well-being findings, we will identify issues more clearly and over time, much more quickly. We will undoubtedly find new ways to work across sectors. And we in government will inevitably develop creative solutions working *with* the communities we exist to support. We will build on strengths and assets. We will be laser-focused on equity: Who is better off? Who is burdened? Who is deciding? We will respond with innovations that will be much more targeted. And finally, we will be able to definitively measure how effective those innovations are—allowing us to modify, scrap, or scale them—for optimal success.

Given its extraordinary potential, well-being should become a goal of all governments. I would argue that it's irresponsible to do anything less.

Afterword

The Future of Well-Being

LAURA D. KUBZANSKY, PHD, MPH
Department of Social and Behavioral Sciences,
Lee Kum Sheung Center for Health and Happiness,
Harvard T.H. Chan School of Public Health, United States

While the concept of well-being has long been of interest to scientists and health practitioners, it often fails to capture attention and resources in the way that disease and death do. The vast majority of health-oriented research focuses on identifying and mitigating problems to reduce disease burden rather than identifying and developing strategies to enhance well-being per se. Discussion and research presented in the current volume make the case for shifting the focus to well-being. However, if we truly want to place well-being at the center of efforts to define and understand population health, we will need a robust *science* of well-being. Theoretical and empirical research across multiple disciplines provides a strong foundation, but this work has been limited by the tendency for academic silos to discourage dialogue, and by the sense that relative to studying suffering, studying well-being is less valuable and less urgent. To advance the science and provide the strongest possible evidence base for practice, future work in this area will benefit from a clear articulation of a well-being approach that goes beyond focusing on the absence of disease and encompasses concepts of positive health.

The insights in this volume recognize the need to bring together work across a range of disciplines, not only to inform the development of effective techniques for measuring well-being, but also to consider the ways a well-being focus can be used to create a healthier society. The perspectives and case studies shared here by Bellagio participants help spark important discussion about best practices in measuring well-being, key issues to consider if we were to adopt well-being as a progress indicator in addition to traditional measures of GDP, and whether and how measuring well-being might affect practice and policy in substantive ways.

A Positive Health Versus Deficit-Based Approach

In the United States, a strong focus on disease rather than health is evident in both medicine and public health, including in the basic science of public health, epidemiology. In the context of medicine, a focus on disease and its absence can be practical as it permits relatively clear assessments of whether a treatment has been successful or if a policy facilitates obtaining treatment (for a more nuanced discussion, see Sartorius [2006]).[1] However, from a population health perspective, a focus on disease, deficits, and problems may limit capacity to understand health in several ways.

First, a disease and deficit focus may result in a highly skewed understanding of what it means to be healthy. Without understanding what optimal health looks like, it will be difficult to identify those conditions that make optimal health more likely at either the individual or population level. Recognizing this problem, in 2010 the American Heart Association proposed a new initiative to promote "cardiovascular health," arguing that without a clear definition of cardiovascular health as a different endpoint from cardiovascular disease, cardiovascular medicine was missing critical insight.[2,3] However, this remains one of the few positive health metrics available to date. Moreover, even when research focuses on positive health outcomes, it can still be dominated by a deficit-based approach in part because processes known to signal or contribute to deterioration are more established. For example, most research considering biological underpinnings or sequelae of well-being examines presence or absence of deteriorative processes like chronic low-level inflammation or elevated blood pressure.[4] Research on biological processes that uniquely contribute to effective functioning (e.g., those invoked with physical activity or with a healthy gut microbiome) is rare.[5]

Second, identifying and evaluating exposures that elevate risk of disease (e.g., poor nutrition, pollution, discrimination), can provide only a limited understanding of the forces that shape health.[6] In fact, research has increasingly demonstrated that the absence of a risk factor or negative attribute (e.g., maltreatment, depression) is not equivalent to the presence of a positive factor (e.g., parental warmth, emotional vitality). For example, in research examining whether facets of positive psychological well-being reduce risk of developing chronic disease among initially healthy populations, the most rigorous studies consistently demonstrate associations that are independent of psychological distress.[7,8] Furthermore, numerous studies suggest positive psychological and social assets (e.g., parental warmth, social integration, optimism) serve as up-stream determinants of more proximal causes of health, including behavior[8-12] and biological function.[13,14] This is consistent with early evidence suggesting that interventions at the individual, organizational, and policy level that enhance psychological well-being may also improve physical health outcomes (e.g., Huffman [2016],[15] Kossek [2019],[16] Peterson [2012],[17] and Thornton [2016][18]). As a result, a recent commentary has called for expanding epidemiologic research to incorporate a "positive epidemiology" focusing on health assets and a broad range of health-related states.[6]

Finally, attention to positive health and well-being may make health promotion and intervention strategies more palatable for individuals, organizations, and communities. A focus on health equity and health disparities often results in highlighting deficits and problems within specific communities, which can be demoralizing and overwhelming. For example, studies routinely point out the higher burden of disease and mortality in blacks, individuals with lower education and income, and other socially disadvantaged groups.[19] Approaches that consider both building assets and mitigating deficits may be more effective than either alone (Fietje and Thomas, chapter 5).

Thus, shifting our frame from one of deficits to one of assets—from one of disease to one of flourishing or well-being—promotes consideration of a different set of questions and expectations. It leads us to ask how we might define optimal functioning (i.e., are there biological measures of thriving) and to consider what are the conditions needed to make this more likely to occur at a population level. It impels us to go beyond simply focusing on the presence or absence of a problem, to solving for how we increase positive health levels within and across populations. This is highly congruent with a health equity framework that seeks to ensure everyone in a population has the opportunity to achieve health. This approach requires not only removing conditions that increase risk of poor health, but also ensuring opportunity to attain resources that promote positive health. At present, we have less understanding of what these resources are. With a well-being approach grounded in health equity, we are compelled to maintain greater focus on such resources and create equity in opportunities to attain them.

The Challenge of Defining Well-Being

If well-being is to be a major target for policy and research,[20] then defining and measuring well-being becomes paramount. The concept of well-being is designed to capture how individuals and communities experience and evaluate their lives, encompassing mental and physical health. To assess these various components, multiple measures have been developed, which can be divided into two domains. The first, objective well-being, includes quantifiable indicators of socio-environmental conditions, such as levels of education, income, safety, community vitality, and democratic engagement. The second, subjective well-being, includes indicators of how individuals assess their own life based on cognitive judgments and affective reactions. Both objective and subjective well-being have been considered in different studies and across disciplines not only as outcomes, but also as predictors.

Moreover, policymakers have begun using these measures to inform policy objectives as well as actions they might take to achieve these objectives. For example, as Tim Ng describes in chapter 9, the New Zealand Treasury has developed the Living Standards Framework, which makes explicit how economic, fiscal, and regulatory activities might be connected with well-being objectives. Guided by the framework, they are working to identify relevant social and economic conditions (i.e., objective well-being) and individual-level experiences (i.e., subjective well-being) that should be measured and monitored. However, as many participants contributing to the discussion in this volume noted, to continue to move research and policy forward effectively, several issues related to the definition of well-being and its measurement need careful attention. These include the importance of using comparable metrics, clearly distinguishing between well-being and conditions that predict well-being, and consistent guidance regarding what types of measures are useful for various endeavors.

Numerous overall well-being indices have been created for the purposes of tracking country-level (or other administrative units') performance with regard to growth and development, as an alternative to GDP (e.g., Stiglitz [2009],[21] United Nations Development Programme [2018][22]). Often including measures of objective and subjective well-being, these indices have also been used to rank countries according to their level of well-being, and to identify policies or other societal attributes that might influence well-being. There are several problems with these indices as currently formulated. First, they lack comparability because components are not uniform across the different indices, and as a result, rankings can differ widely. Perhaps of greater concern is that objective well-being is *defined by* factors that create conditions under which attaining subjective well-being is more or less likely. For example, objective well-being is often characterized according to levels of education, poverty rates, labor market security, aspects of the community, and participation in leisure or cultural activities in a given society. However, these same factors are also considered social determinants of health.[23] We will not answer the call to identify root causes of well-being (Acharya and Plough, Introduction), if the exposure (i.e., social determinants) and the outcome (i.e., well-being) are comprised of the same elements. As noted by Bradshaw et al.,[24] "too many indicators in the objective domains [of well-being] are about well-becoming rather than well-being."

I would suggest we no longer use the term "objective well-being," but rather consider the elements of objective well-being as social determinants of subjective well-being.

Reframing the idea of "objective well-being" as social determinants, or a set of conditions that affect the likelihood of achieving subjective well-being and positive health, could have important implications for both research and policies designed to improve population health. For example, with current terminology, countries with higher levels of income and education are characterized as having high (objective) well-being, implying that more individuals in that country have attained high levels of (subjective) well-being per se. This may or may not be the case, depending on other conditions and factors. However, it could be fair to assume that there is increased likelihood that more of the population will achieve positive health in these countries, and perhaps greater health equity as a result. Once we separate social determinants from subjective well-being, this assumption can be tested empirically and contribute to an evidence base that can inform policy and practice. Moreover, this separation also makes it possible to disentangle correlation from causation, identifying those conditions that truly contribute to positive health versus those that simply travel alongside of causal factors. Ultimately, such information can point policymakers to strategies that are more targeted and effective for improving population health.

Important measurement issues remain even when considering only the domain of subjective well-being. There is often confusion about how it is defined and assessed. As reviewed by Carol Graham in chapter 3, relevant psychological states fall within three subdomains, including hedonic, eudaimonic, and evaluative well-being, and a variety of strategies can be taken to obtain high-quality measures used to characterize these states. While there are a number of overviews of the many subjective well-being measures that are available,[25-27] few provide guidance on which measures to use for what purpose. Moreover, despite a strong understanding of methodologic factors that enhance (or detract from) the quality of items used in such measures, conceptual confusion remains with regard to distinguishing *subjective well-being* from two other related concepts, *psychological well-being* and *flourishing*. Absent clear conceptual definitions and recommendations and given the numerous measures available, organizations or studies that might want to measure or monitor subjective well-being often feel paralyzed. Some guidance is needed if we want to make assessment of well-being more effective, widespread, and accessible.

In fact, although many organizations, and particularly the Organisation for Economic Co-operation and Development, have suggested potential well-being indicators, unlike with other health outcomes (e.g., the American Heart Association convenes strategic planning committees to set national goals for cardiovascular health promotion and disease reduction), there is still a great deal of confusion as to which indicators to use when, and it remains unclear as to whether there is a single organization or body that is responsible (or viewed as the authority) for setting standards for how best to achieve well-being. To begin to fill this gap, a multidisciplinary group of experts in well-being recently published a detailed discussion addressing how subjective well-being may be distinguished from related concepts, and also proposing a set of recommendations for choosing well-being measures for use in research and practice.[28] While they are not definitive, by leveraging the strongest measures available and taking account of real-world constraints individuals might encounter when trying to use these measures, these recommendations provide some guidance to facilitate continued progress. Different measurement approaches will be required depending on whether a given measure will be used for tracking and surveillance, for research seeking to evaluate determinants of well-being, or for research evaluating effects of subjective well-being on other outcomes. Thus, specific measures are proposed for different purposes, including for assessing well-being in government surveys versus multi-use cohort studies versus studies of psychological well-being or flourishing.

Several other issues related to measuring well-being across countries, over time, and across the life course are worth mentioning. First, with some notable exceptions (e.g., the United Kingdom), few countries routinely collect data on subjective well-being. As pointed out earlier in this volume (Prah Ruger, chapter 1), we cannot see what is not measured, and, if we care about subjective well-being, then we need to make it visible. Second, most subjective well-being measures are designed for adults. Until recently, research in childhood has largely relied on a heterogenous set of measures that do not correspond clearly to domains defined for adulthood.[24] While recent work provides more guidance on measuring subjective well-being in later childhood and adolescence,[29] when and whether younger children can report on their own subjective well-being remains unclear. Moreover, the conditions likely to predict child and adult subjective well-being may not completely overlap. When considering subjective well-being at different life stages, investigators will need to consider at least some socio-environmental conditions that are specific to that life stage.

Future Directions and Key Outstanding Questions

Throughout this volume, authors have identified potential challenges with applying a well-being approach to advance equity. A critical issue is whether facets of subjective well-being are universal or if they can only be understood according to the cultural contexts within which people make meaning. A related question is whether similar well-being measures are equally valid in different populations. In addition, we need to distinguish whether we are measuring conditions that promote or impede individuals' capacity to flourish, specific facets of psychological functioning, or other aspects of lived experience. These distinctions are important because different facets of well-being may vary in level of susceptibility to specific environmental conditions.

Also important will be to define optimal functioning and evaluate the role of health assets separately from that of risk factors. Given the growing body of research suggesting facets of subjective well-being predict and precede physical health,[8,30] systematic monitoring of appropriate measures of subjective well-being in a population might provide an early-warning sign of physical health trends. However, separating measures of psychological functioning (e.g., subjective well-being) from more comprehensive measures that capture both psychological and physical functioning (e.g., flourishing) is critical to conducting nuanced study of the inter-relationships between psychological and physical health.

A detailed social epidemiology of subjective well-being does not exist. Currently, data regarding the role of social structural factors are largely from observational studies providing a snapshot of how individuals are functioning at a single point in time, limiting causal inference. Relying primarily on these types of studies, the most recent World Happiness Report identified six factors posited to influence subjective well-being at a country level, including GDP per capita, social support, healthy life expectancy, freedom to make life choices, generosity, and freedom from corruption.[31] Experimental research providing some evidence of causality was available only for generosity and social support.[32-34] There are true methodological challenges with this type of research. For example, manipulating certain factors of interest (e.g., GDP per capita) to address questions of causality may not be ethical or possible. However, similar limitations have been solved in other research domains, and these solutions can be applied to the study of well-being.[6]

Conclusion

Our current state of knowledge on the distribution and determinants of well-being, as well as effects of well-being approaches, is limited less by capacity for research in this area than by a dominant intellectual framework in public health and medicine whose central focus is disease and the causes of pathology.[5] To identify, understand, and promote conditions required for human well-being we need to expand this framework or shift the current paradigm from a focus on deficits to a focus on assets and positive health outcomes. In fact, this is a core idea behind the Culture of Health approach pursued by the Robert Wood Johnson Foundation and others: "For too long, we have defined being healthy as simply not being sick. . . . After decades of focus on the health care system, we have come to recognize that complex social factors have a powerful influence on our well-being. We see more clearly than ever that to improve the nation's health, we must engage all sectors to improve population health, well-being, and equity."[35]

Existing tools and measures can take us quite far in addressing critical outstanding issues and making visible experiences and conditions that are currently invisible. No doubt there are some questions for which we do not yet have the tools or methods to address. In fact, Carol Graham and others in this volume reiterate the importance of developing strong measures but also caution that it will be important to accept some level of uncertainty regarding the quality of our measures in order to continue moving forward with measuring and monitoring well-being. But consider this: four decades ago it did not seem possible to sequence the genome and use that information to find the genetic roots of disease and develop treatment. After this endeavor was declared a national (and international) priority, the Human Genome Project was launched and the genome was successfully sequenced. Thus, experience suggests that with sufficient support and attention to issues of positive health, the capacity to address them will follow.

Conclusion

Momentum for Change but Challenges Persist

ALONZO L. PLOUGH, PHD, MPH, MA

*Chief Science Officer and Vice President, Research-Evaluation-Learning
Robert Wood Johnson Foundation, United States*

The Bellagio convening took place over two a year ago, and global interest in a well-being approach to address inequity and improve life chances continues to grow. Katrín Jakobsdóttir, Iceland's prime minister, recently called for "an alternative future based on well-being and inclusive growth."[1] This plea—prompted, she says, in large part to curtail environmental devastation and the implications of climate change for human survival—puts Iceland in good company with other countries that have taken a well-being approach to policy and budgeting. By redefining progress to include not only economic strength, but also people's quality of life and ability to create the futures they want, Jakobsdóttir and other leaders are charting a course for a more sustainable and equitable future.

There are similar headlines from around the globe: As presented in this volume, New Zealand announced a well-being budget that prioritizes a low-emissions economy, advances skills and opportunities, reduces child poverty, and supports mental health.[2] Scotland's first minister, Nicola Sturgeon, made "the case for a much broader definition of what it means to be successful as a country, as a society," calling for modern economies to put more resources into mental health, child care and parental leave, and green energy.[3] Gus O'Donnell, cabinet secretary to three U.K. prime ministers, said that achieving well-being, not economic growth, should be the primary aim of government spending.[4]

Here in the United States, in Santa Monica, California—as Julia Rusk's commentary describes—city government declared more than five years ago that its purpose is to improve the well-being of its residents.

There are other examples, mostly local, around the United States where a well-being framework is catalyzing community and governmental action.

However, as a nation, we continue to make critical public policy decisions with an imbalanced focus on growth and consumption. A recent domestic headline, the week before Iceland's, was a new report in the *Journal of the American Medical Association* (*JAMA*) about a spike in deaths among young and middle-age adults.[5] While the average global life expectancy has been steadily on the rise, this report by RWJF grantees Steven Woolf and Heidi Schoomaker at Virginia Commonwealth University showed that average life expectancy in the United States has decreased for three consecutive years.

The report pointed to suicide, drug overdoses, liver disease, and dozens of other causes. Bellagio participant Carol Graham at Brookings Institution and a professor at the University of Maryland and others have dubbed these "diseases of despair," preceded by years of isolation, worry, and hopelessness—conditions we would see if we prioritized and were paying attention to well-being indicators. These early clues might allow us to take action way before long-term negative health outcomes take root.

In addition to the *JAMA* report, other work by our grantees singles out lack of nutritious food and places to be active, relentless tobacco marketing, inadequate early childhood education and family support, social isolation and lack of belonging, and gaps in housing, education, infrastructure, jobs, and other social factors that determine our ability to be healthy, or not. COVID-19, which continues to spread across the United States and around the world as this book goes to press, has sharply illuminated these inequitable conditions. Rates of infection and complications from the virus are markedly higher in communities of color, immigrant communities, and other groups that live with higher rates of air pollution, spotty health coverage, persistent health inequities, and lack of paid leave or a financial safety net to follow "stay home" public health orders. This virus has laid bare a system that was already deeply flawed. As we recover, prepare for potential future outbreaks, and eventually rebuild, it is imperative that we prioritize equitable well-being as the ultimate goal. This would dramatically shift attention and investment on these issues, as demonstrated by the new budgets coming out of New Zealand and other countries (and mirrored in the reality of new Zealand's currently exceptionally low COVID-19 mortality rate).

This book offers evidence that a well-being movement is gaining momentum, and shows tremendous need and opportunity for further exploration and scaling.

While this movement remains nascent in the United States, there are multiple opportunities to accelerate the pace of change. It is a tangible reality with bright spots at all levels and in diverse places, going beyond a theory or a new set of measures. There are significant challenges, but also opportunities to move from a set of experiments and time-limited innovations to sustainable changes across societies that improve well-being. This requires both urgency and long-term thinking; the work will advance through rapid experimentation and a commitment to generational change. And equity must be at the core of this change.

What has RWJF has been doing on well-being since Bellagio?

1. Research to explore the role of hope, flourishing, and other well-being indicators.
2. Exploration of well-being indicators to incorporate within our own measures, as well as discussions with the Centers for Disease Control and Prevention and others about how to integrate well-being indicators into national measures, with emphasis on addition of subjective measures.
3. Early conversations about how to shift narratives and mindsets to align with and advance a well-being approach.
4. Ongoing learning from innovators at the local and national levels, including a learning trip to Bhutan.
5. Considerations of how to advance well-being approaches and outcomes among specific sectors.

We hope this book adds to both the science and the actions to advance well-being, and provides instructive examples and questions to consider in your own work.

- **For policymakers and local and national leaders:** Consider ways you can center decision-making, evaluation, and goal setting on well-being measures. Look to the Organisation for Economic Co-operation and Development's Better Life Index indicators as a starting point.
- **For news media:** Tell the stories of efforts to advance well-being, and look for new measures, beyond economics-only, to use in your reporting. Look at Solutions Journalism Network for inspiration.
- **For practitioners across sectors:** Consider how your plans, actions, and evaluation of progress can broaden to include indicators of well-being. Follow Wellbeing Economy Alliance for examples and resources.
- **For academics and researchers in economics, public health, and other fields:** Explore the evolving field of well-being, reflect on the cautions and methodological challenges suggested in Laura Kubzansky's commentary, and help build the body of evidence for a well-being approach.

Thank you to the contributors to the rich dialogue presented in this volume, and to the global community that will expand and adapt these ideas to their own historical and local contexts. We remain committed to learning along with you.

BELLAGIO CONVENING PARTICIPANT LIST

*The Robert Wood Johnson Foundation Well-Being Convening
at Rockefeller Bellagio Conference Center*

Participants

Tarek Abu Fakhr, Adviser, National Program for Happiness and Wellbeing, United Arab Emirates

Mao Amis, Founder and Executive Director, African Centre for a Green Economy, South Africa

David Bornstein, B.Com, MA, Co-Founder and CEO, Solutions Journalism Network; Writer, *New York Times*, United States

Sir Harry Burns, Professor, Global Public Health, University of Strathclyde, Scotland

Anita Chandra, DrPH, MPH, Vice President and Director, RAND Social and Economic Well-Being, RAND Corporation, United States

Kee-Seng Chia, Founding Dean and Professor, Saw Swee Hock School of Public Health, National University of Singapore

Mallika Dutt, MIA, JD, Founder and Director, Inter-Connected, United States

Carrie Exton, DPhil, Head of Section, Monitoring Well-Being and Progress, Statistics and Data Directorate, Organisation for Economic Co-operation and Development, France

Nils Fietje, PhD, Research Officer, Regional Office for Europe, World Health Organization, Denmark

Walter Flores, PhD, Executive Director, Center for the Study of Equity and Governance in Health Systems, Guatemala

Rita Giacaman, Professor, Institute of Community and Public Health, Birzeit University, Palestine

Carol Graham, AB, MA, DPhil, Leo Pasvolsky Senior Fellow, the Brookings Institution; College Park Professor, the University of Maryland, United States

Danny Graham, QC, CEO, Engage Nova Scotia, Canada

Dr. Shariha Khalid Erichsen, MSc, MBChB, MRCS, Managing Partner, Mission & Co., Southeast Asia

Dr. Julia Kim, MD, MSc, FRCPS (C), Program Director, GNH Centre Bhutan

Dr. Éloi Laurent, Senior Economist, Sciences Po Centre for Economic Research, France; Visiting Professor, Stanford University, United States

Gora Mboup, President and CEO, Global Observatory linking Research to Action (GORA) Corp, United States and Senegal

Romlie Mokak, BSocSci, PG Dip Sp Ed, Commissioner, Productivity Commission, Australian Government; (former) CEO, Lowitja Institute, Australia

José Molinas Vega, PhD, Chief Economist, Development Institute; (former) Minister-Secretary of Planning for Economic and Social Development, Republic of Paraguay

Dr. Claire A. Nelson, Lead Futurist, the Futures Forum, United States and the Caribbean

Tim Ng, Deputy Secretary and Chief Economic Adviser, the New Zealand Treasury

Anita Rajan, BA, BEd, MBA, CEO, Tata STRIVE; Vice President, Tata Community Initiatives Trust, Tata Group, India

Jennifer Prah Ruger, PhD, MSc, MSL, MA, Amartya Sen Professor of Health Equity, Economics and Policy, School of Social Policy and Practice and Perelman School of Medicine, University of Pennsylvania, United States

Katherine Trebeck, BA, PhD, Knowledge and Policy Lead, Wellbeing Economy Alliance, Scotland

Nancy Wildfeir-Field, President, GBCHealth, United States and Africa

Liz Zeidler, Chief Executive, Happy City, United Kingdom

Convening Hosts

Richard E. Besser, MD, President and CEO, Robert Wood Johnson Foundation, United States

Alonzo L. Plough, PhD, MPH, MA, Chief Science Officer and Vice President of Research-Evaluation-Learning, Robert Wood Johnson Foundation, United States

Karabi Acharya, ScD, MHS, Director, Global Ideas for U.S. Solutions, Robert Wood Johnson Foundation, United States

Convening Designers and Facilitators

Eric Friedenwald-Fishman, Creative Director/Founder, Metropolitan Group, United States

Jennifer Messenger, Executive Vice President, Metropolitan Group, United States

Convening Project Manager

Trené Hawkins, Program Associate, Robert Wood Johnson Foundation, United States

ACKNOWLEDGMENTS

ALONZO L. PLOUGH, EDITOR IN CHIEF

Chief Science Officer and Vice President of Research-Evaluation-Learning, Robert Wood Johnson Foundation, United States

This book is the product of a compelling week with 32 leaders and thinkers, but it represents a much more extensive conversation. From the introductions and exploration that led to the gathering, to the conversations and actions that have happened since, this is truly an ongoing learning journey. We owe our gratitude to many contributors.

Our editorial review group
Sandro Galea, MD, MPH, DrPH, Dean and Robert A. Knox Professor at Boston University School of Public Health
Sherry Glied, MA, PhD, Dean and Professor, New York University's Robert F. Wagner Graduate School of Public Service
Chad Zimmerman, former Senior Editor, Oxford University Press

Editorial team at the Robert Wood Johnson Foundation
Karabi Acharya, Director, Global Ideas for U.S. Solutions
Kristin Silvani, Learning Coordinator

Project team at Metropolitan Group
Jennifer Messenger, lead editor
Matt Baer
Tovar Cerulli
Elizabeth Friedenwald
Eric Friedenwald-Fishman
Rob Sassor

Writers
  Lori De Milto
  Leila Fiester
  Susan Parker

And of course to all of the participants who joined us in Bellagio, who are listed in the previous section—particularly those who prepared papers and case studies for the gathering and for this book.

REFERENCES

Foreword

1. World Health Organization. *Who We Are: Frequently Asked Questions. www.who.int/about/ who-we-are/frequently-asked-questions.* Accessed September 17, 2019.

Introduction

1. Sturgeon N. (2019, July). *Why Governments Should Prioritize Well-Being.* TED Summit 2019. *www.ted.com/talks/nicola_sturgeon_why_governments_should_priori-tize_well_being? language=en.* Accessed September 22, 2019.
2. World Economic Forum. (2019, June 24). *Jacinda Ardern: Politics and Economics to Focus on Empathy, Kindness and Well-Being. youtube.com/watch?v=GqzlFffL0W4.* Accessed September 22, 2019.

Chapter 1

1. Piketty T, Goldhammer A. *Capital in the Twenty-First Century.* Cambridge, Mass: The Belknap Press of Harvard University Press; 2014.
2. Ostrom E. Beyond Markets and States: Polycentric Governance of Complex Economic Systems. *American Economic Review.* 2010;100(3):641–672.
3. Laurent E. *Measuring Tomorrow: Accounting for Well-Being, Resilience, and Sustainability in the Twenty-First Century.* Princeton, NJ: Princeton University Press; 2018.
4. Motesharrei S, Rivas J, Kalnay E. Human and Nature Dynamics (HANDY): Modeling Inequality and Use of Resources in the Collapse or Sustainability of Societies. *Ecological Economics.* 2014;101:90–102.
5. Gough I. *Heat, Greed and Human Need: Climate Change, Capitalism and Sustainable Wellbeing.* Cheltenham, UK: Edward Elgar; 2017.
6. People's Agreement of Cochabamba. World People's Conference on Climate Change and the Rights of Mother Earth. April 22, 2010, Cochabamba, Bolivia. *pwccc.wordpress.com/2010/ 04/24/peoples-agreement/.* Accessed October 17, 2019.

7. Encyclical Letter Laudato Si' of The Holy Father Francis on Care for our Common Home, May 24, 2015. *w2.vatican.va/content/francesco/en/encyclicals/documents/papafrancesco_20150524_enciclica-laudato-si.html*. Accessed October 17, 2019.

8. World Health Organization. 10 Facts on Health Inequities and Their Causes. April 2017. *www.who.int/features/factfiles/health_inequities/en/*. Accessed October 17, 2019.

9. Organisation for Economic Co-operation and Development. Perspectives on Global Development: Social Cohesion in a Shifting World. Paris; 2012.

10. Carey T. Defining Australian Indigenous Wellbeing: Do We Really Want the Answer? Implication for Policy and Practice. *Psychotherapy and Politics International.* 2013;11(3):182–194.

11. Burns J, Hull G, Lefko-Everett K, Njoleza L. Defining Social Cohesion. Cape Town: SALDRU, UCT; 2018. (SALDRU Working Paper Number 216.)

Chapter 2

1. Xie J, Sreenivasan S, Korniss G, Zhang W, Lim C, Szymanski BK. Social Consensus through the Influence of Committed Minorities. [Abstract]. *Physical Review E.* 2011;84:011130. *journals.aps.org/pre/abstract/10.1103/PhysRevE.84.011130*. Accessed August 15, 2019.

Chapter 3

(References Provided by Author.)

1. Graham C, Laffan K, Pinto S. Well-Being in Metrics and Policy. *Science.* 2018;362:6412.

2. Case A, Deaton, A. Mortality and Morbidity in the 21st Century. *Brookings Papers on Economic Activity. Spring 2017.* March 23, 2017. *https://www.brookings.edu/bpea-articles/mortality and-morbidity-in-the-21st-century/*. Accessed September 22, 2019.

3. Graham C, Pinto S. Unequal Hopes and Lives in the U.S.: The Role of Race, Place, and Premature Mortality. *Journal of Population Economics.* 2019;32(2):665–733.

4. Trust for America's Health (TFAH). *Pain in the Nation: The Drug, Alcohol, and Suicide Crisis and the Need for a National Resilience Strategy. Issue Report.* Washington, D.C.: 2017.

5. O'Connor K, Graham C. Longer, More Optimistic Lives: Historic Optimism and Life Expectancy in the United States. *STATEC Working Papers.* Luxembourg: July 2018.

6. Ifcher J, Zarghamee H, Graham C. Local Neighbors as Positives, Regional Neighbors as Negatives: Competing Channels in the Relationship Between Others' Income, Health, and Happiness. *Journal of Health Economics.* 2018;57:263–276.

7. Graham C. Happiness and Health: Lessons—and Questions—for Policy. *Health Affairs.* 2008;27(2):72–87.

8. Eberstadt N. *Men without Work: America's Invisible Crisis.* West Conshohocken, Penn.: Templeton; 2016.

9. Graham C, Zhou S, Zhang J. Happiness and Health in China: The Paradox of Progress. *World Development.* 2017;96:231–244.

10. Stone A, Mackie C. *Subjective Well-Being: Measuring Happiness, Suffering, and Other Dimensions of Human Experience.* Washington, D.C.: National Research Council of the National Academies; 2013. Retrieved from *http://www.nap.edu/catalog.php?record_id=18548*

11. Graham C, Nikolova N. Bentham or Aristotle in the Development Process? An Empirical Investigation of Capabilities and Subjective Well-Being. *World Development.* 2015;68:163–179.

12. Graham C. *Happiness around the World: The Paradox of Happy Peasants and Miserable Millionaires.* Oxford: Oxford University Press; 2009.

13. Graham C. *Happiness for All? Unequal Hopes and Lives in Pursuit of the American Dream.* Princeton, N.J.: Princeton University Press; 2017.

14. Graham C, Eggers A, Sukhtankar S. Does Happiness Pay? An Initial Exploration Based on Panel Data from Russia. *Journal of Economic Behavior & Organization.* 2004;55:319–342.

15. De Neve J-E, Oswald A. Estimating the Effects of Life Satisfaction and Positive Affect on Later Outcomes Using Sibling Data. *Proceedings of the National Academy of Sciences of the United States.* 2012;109(49):19953–19958.

16. De Neve J-E, Diener E, Tay L, Xuereb C. The Objective Benefits of Subjective Well Being. In: Helliwell J, Layard J, Sachs, J, eds. *World Happiness Report II.* New York: Earth Institute, Columbia University; 2013:54–74.

17. City of Santa Monica. Communicating the Wellbeing of a City with Santa Monica. *https:// designmattersatartcenter.org/proj/wellbeing-santa-monica/.* Accessed September 18, 2019.

18. What Works Well-Being. www.whatworkswellbeing.org/. Accessed September 18, 2019.

19. Office for National Statistics. Personal Well-Being in the UK QMI. *www.ons.gov.uk/ peoplepopulationandcommunity/wellbeing/methodologies/personalwellbeingintheukqmi.* Accessed September 18, 2019.

20. Graham C, Pettinato S, Frustrated Achievers: Winners, Losers, and Subjective Well-Being in the New Market Economies. *Journal of Development Studies.* April 2002;38(4).

21. Native American Connections. *www.nativeconnections.org.* Accessed September 18, 2019.

22. Graham C, Juneau J, Pinto S. *The Geography of Desperation in America.* 2017. The Brookings Institution. *www.brookings.edu/research/the-geography-of-desperation-in-america*

23. Graham C, Ruiz-Pozuelo J. Does Hope Lead to Better Futures: Evidence from a Survey of the Life Choices of Young Adults in Peru. *Global Views,* #10, The Brookings Institution, March 2019. *www.brookings.edu/wp-content/uploads/2018/03/hope_better_futures_working_ paper11.pdf*

Chapter 4

1. Bureau of Economic Analysis, U.S. Department of Commerce. Gross Domestic Product. *www.bea.gov/data/gdp/gross-domestic-product.* Accessed September 18, 2019.

2. Lee Kum Sheung Center for Health and Happiness. Repository of Positive Psychological Well-Being Scales. *www.hsph.harvard.edu/health-happiness/repository-of-positive-psychological-well-being-scales.* Accessed September 18, 2019.

3. Office for National Statistics. Personal and Economic Well-Being in the UK: April 2019. *www. ons.gov.uk/peoplepopulationandcommunity/wellbeing/bulletins/personalandeconomicwellbeing intheuk/april2019#dashboard-of-well-being-indicators.* Accessed September 18, 2019.

4. John F. Kennedy Presidential Library. Robert F. Kennedy, Remarks at the University of Kansas, March 18, 1968. *www.jfklibrary.org/learn/about-jfk/the-kennedy-family/robert-f-kennedy/robert-f-kennedy-speeches/remarks-at-the-university-of-kansas-march-18-1968.* Accessed September 28, 2019.

5. Organisation for Economic Co-operation and Development (OECD). *www. oecdbetterlifeindex.org.* Accessed September 28, 2019.

6. Organisation for Economic Co-operation and Development (OECD) Statistical Commission. (2014). *Some National, Regional and International Efforts and Practices in the Measurement of Sustainable Development and Human Well-Being.* February 2014. *https:// unstats.un.org/unsd/broaderprogress/pdf/BG-FOC-Broader%20measures-Practices%20on%20 broader%20measures%20of%20progress.pdf.* Accessed September 28, 2019.

7. European Social Survey. Frequently Asked Questions. *www.europeansocialsurvey.org/about/ faq.html.* Accessed September 28, 2019.

8. Centre for Bhutan Studies and GNH Research. (2015, November 3). *Largest Ever Conference on Gross National Happiness Held in Paro Bhutan, for the 60th Birthday Celebrations of Bhutan's*

4th King, the Architect of GNH. [Press Release]. *www.grossnationalhappiness.com/conference/2015-gnh-conference/press-release/.* Accessed September 28, 2019.

9. Centre for Bhutan Studies and GNH Research. 2015 GNH Survey Report. *www.grossnationalhappiness.com.* Accessed September 28, 2019.

10. Oxford Poverty & Human Development Initiative (OPHI). Bhutan's Gross National Happiness Index. *https://ophi.org.uk/policy/national-policy/gross-national-happiness-index* Accessed September 28, 2019.

11. Charlton E. New Zealand Has Unveiled Its First "Well-Being" Budget. World Economic Forum. *www.weforum.org/agenda/2019/05/new-zealand-is-publishing-its-first-well-being-budget.* Accessed December 10, 2019.

12. Halverson JR. *Why Story Is Not Narrative.* Center for Strategic Communication at Arizona State University. December 8, 2011. *https://csc.asu.edu/2011/12/08/why-story-is-not-narrative*

13. Frank AW. *Letting Stories Breathe.* Chicago: University of Chicago Press; 2010.

14. Fisher WR. Narration as a Human Communication Paradigm: The Case of Public Moral Argument. *Communication Monographs.* 1984;51:1–22.

15. Bruner J. The Narrative Construction of Reality. *Critical Inquiry.* 1991;18(1);1–22.

16. The Narrative Initiative. *https://narrativeinitiative.org/blog/narrative-change-a-working-definition-and-related-terms.* Accessed November 19, 2019.

17. Cameron WB. *Informal Sociology: A Casual Introduction to Sociological Thinking.* New York: Random House; 1963.

18. Organisation for Economic Co-operation and Development (OECD). OECD Guidelines on Measuring Subjective Well-Being. Paris: OECD Publishing; 2013.

19. Deaton A. Income, Health, and Well-Being around the World: Evidence from the Gallup World Poll. *Journal of Economic Perspectives.* 2008;22(2):53–72. Cited in Conceição P, Romina B. Measuring Subjective Wellbeing: A Summary Review of the Literature. (2008). *https://pdfs.semanticscholar.org/1772/72a223411959e11966369c04b6f88a7b07c8.pdf.* Accessed November 19, 2019.

20. Conceição P, Romina B. Measuring Subjective Wellbeing: A Summary Review of the Literature. 2008. *https://pdfs.semanticscholar.org/1772/72a223411959e11966369c04b6f88a7b07c8.pdf.* Accessed November 19, 2019.

21. Stiglitz J. Towards a Better Measure of Well-Being. *Financial Times.* September 13, 2009. *www.ft.com/content/95b492a8-a095-11de-b9ef-00144feabdc0*

22. Oxfam Humankind Index: The New Measure of Scotland's Prosperity, Second Results. June 2013. *www.issuelab.org/resource/oxfam-humankind-index-the-new-measure-of-scotlands-prosperity-second-results.html*

23. Cultural Survival. The Issues. *www.culturalsurvival.org/issues.* Accessed November 19, 2019.

24. US Department of Transportation. Guidance on Treatment of the Value of Preventing Fatalities and Injuries in Preparing Economic Analysis. Revised Departmental Guidance 2016. August 8, 2016. *www.transportation.gov/sites/dot.gov/files/docs/2016%20Revised%20Value%20of%20a%20Statistical%20Life%20Guidance.pdf.* Accessed November 19, 2019.

25. Happy City. Invest in Happy. *www.happycity.org.uk.* Accessed November 19, 2019.

26. Letter from the Acting Secretary of Commerce Transmitting in Response to Senate Resolution No. 220 (72D CONG.) A Report on National Income, 1929–32. January 4, 1934. *https://fraser.stlouisfed.org/files/docs/publications/natincome_1934/19340104_nationalinc.pdf*

Chapter 5

(References Provided by Author.)

1. Coyle D. *GDP: A Brief but Affectionate History.* Princeton, N.J.: Princeton University Press; 2014.

2. Stiglitz J, Sen A, Fitoussi J-P. Report of the Commission on the Measurement of Economic Performance and Social Progress. 2009. *http://ec.europa.eu/eurostat/documents/118025/ 118123/Fitoussi+Commission+report*. Accessed July 4, 2018.

3. Sen A. Capability and Well-Being. In: Nussbaum M, Sen A, eds. *The Quality of Life*. Oxford: Clarendon Press; 1993;30–54.

4. Ryan RM, Deci E. On Happiness and Human Potentials: A Review of Research on Hedonic and Eudaimonic Well-Being. *Annual Review of Psychology*. 2001;52:1069–1081.

5. Devine J, White SC. Religion, Politics and the Everyday Moral Order in Bangladesh. *Journal of Contemporary Asia*. 2013;43(1):127–147.

6. Jardine B. The Origins of Happiness. *Limn*. March 2016. *https://limn.it/issues/the-total-archive*. Accessed June 24, 2018.

7. White S. Relational Wellbeing: Re-Centering the Politics of Happiness, Policy and the Self. *Policy and Politics*. 2017;4592:121–136.

8. Lyon A. *The Fifth Wave*. Edinburgh: Scottish Council Foundation; 2003.

9. Hanlon P, Carlisle S, Hannah M, Reilly D, Lyon A. Making the Case for a "Fifth Wave" in Public Health. *Public Health*. 2011;125:30–36.

10. Davies SC, Winpenny E, Ball S, Fowler T, Robin J, Nolte E. For Debate: A New Wave in Public Health Improvement. *The Lancet*. 2014;384:1889–1895.

11. WPP. Viral Video Prompts Smokers to Quit. 2014. *www.wpp.com/wppgov/storage/ourwork/ casestudies/o/ogilvy-smoking-kid*. Accessed July 10, 2019.

12. Foreman, M. Hearts and Minds: How the Marriage Equality Movement Won Over the American Public. *Nonprofit Quarterly*. June 27, 2016. *https://nonprofitquarterly.org/ hearts-minds-marriage-equality-movement-won-american-public*. Accessed September 19, 2019.

13. New Tactics in Human Rights. Rewriting Traditional Stories to Gain a Gender-Sensitive Perspective. *www.newtactics.org*. Accessed July 15, 2019.

14. Routray P, Schmidt WP, Boisson S, Clasen T, Jenkins MW. Socio-Cultural and Behavioural Factors Constraining Latrine Adoption in Rural Coastal Odisha: An Exploratory Qualitative Study. *BMC Public Health*. 2015;15:880.

15. World Health Organization. *The European Health Report 2015, Targets and Beyond—Reaching New Frontiers in Evidence*. Geneva: WHO; 2015.

16. Chase E, Walker R. Constructing Reality?: The "Discursive Truth" of Poverty in Britain and How It Frames the Experience of Shame. In: Chase E, Bantebya-Kyomuhendo G, eds. *Poverty and Shame: Global Experiences*. Oxford: Oxford University Press; 2015:256–270.

17. Loera-González J. Authorised Voices in the Construction of Wellbeing Discourses: A Reflective Ethnographic Experience in Northern Mexico. In: White S, Blackmore C, eds. *Cultures of Wellbeing: Method, Place, Policy*. London: Palgrave Macmillan; 2015;240–259.

18. Dutta M. *Neoliberal Health Organizing: Communication, Meaning and Politics*. Abingdon: Taylor and Francis; 2015.

19. Cooke B, Kothari U. The Case for Participation as Tyranny. In: Cooke B, Kothari U, eds. *Participation: The New Tyranny?* London: Zed Books; 2001.

20. Greenhalgh T. *Cultural Contexts of Health: The Use of Narrative Research in the Health Sector*. Copenhagen: WHO Regional Office for Europe; 2016.

21. Hinchliffe S, Jackson MA, Wyatt K, et al. Healthy Publics: Enabling Cultures and Environments for Health. *Palgrave Communications*. 2018;57.

22. White S. Introduction: The Many Faces of Wellbeing. In: White S, Blackmore C, eds. *Cultures of Wellbeing: Method, Place, Policy*. London: Palgrave Macmillan; 2015;1–44.

23. Durie R, Wyatt K. Connecting Communities and Complexity: A Case Study in Creating the Conditions for Transformational Change. *Critical Public Health*. 2013;23:174–187.

24. Stuteley H, Stead J. From Isolation to Transformation with C2. *www.c2connectingcommunities. co.uk/wp-content/uploads/2016/10/From_Isolation_to_Transformation_with_C2.pdf.* Accessed September 20, 2019.

25. Thomas PN. Contentious Actions and Communication for Social Change: The Public Hearing (Jan Sunwai) as Process. *Journal of Communication.* 2017;67:719–732.

Chapter 6

1. David Foster Wallace. Transcription of the 2005 Commencement Address. May 21, 2005. *https://web.ics.purdue.edu/~drkelly/DFWKenyonAddress2005.pdf*

2. Bruner J. The Narrative Construction of Reality. *Critical Inquiry.* 1991;18(1):1–22.

3. The Narrative Initiative. *https://narrativeinitiative.org/*

4. Davidson B. *Narrative Change and the Open Society Public Health Program.* 2016 *http:// askjustice.org/wp-content/uploads/2016/07/20160711_Narrative-change-paper-1.pdf*

5. Delalande N. Piketty in Paris: Why Don't Popular Economic Ideas Become Policy? *Dissent.* Fall 2014. *www.dissentmagazine.org/article/piketty-in-paris.* Accessed November 19, 2019.

6. Kirkus Review. *Top Incomes in France in the Twentieth Century.* May 8, 2018. *www.kirkusreviews. com/book-reviews/thomas-piketty/top-incomes-in-france-in-the-twentieth-century*

7. Piketty T, Goldhammer A. *Capital in the Twenty-First Century.* Cambridge Mass.: The Belknap Press of Harvard University Press; 2014.

8. Fowler JH, Christakis NA. Dynamic Spread of Happiness in a Large Social Network: Longitudinal Analysis over 20 Years in the Framingham Heart Study. *British Medical Journal.* 2008;337:a2338.

9. Engage Nova Scotia. *The Nova Scotia Quality of Life Initiative.* [YouTube video.] June 19, 2018. *www.youtube.com/watch?v=vKaxb06LIx4&t=1s*

10. Scottish Government. Scotland Performs. *www2.gov.scot/About/Performance/scotPerforms/ outcome/childfamilies*

11. Schwartz SH. Basic Individual Values: Sources and Consequences. In: Sander D, Brosch T, eds. *Handbook of Value* (pp. 63–84). Oxford: Oxford University Press; 2015. Cited in Schwartz SH, Sortheix FM. Values and Subjective Well-Being. In: Diener E, Oishi S, Tay L, eds. *Handbook of Well-Being.* Salt Lake City: DEF Publishers; 2018.

12. Schwartz SH, Sortheix FM. Values and subjective well-being. In: Diener E, Oishi S, Tay L, eds. *Handbook of Well-Being.* Salt Lake City: DEF Publishers; 2018.

13. Borunda A. See How a Warmer World Primed California for Large Fires. *National Geographic.* November 15, 2018. *www.nationalgeographic.com/environment/2018/11/climate-change-california-wildfire*

14. Andrews RG. Flash Floods Threaten More People Than Thought, as Ice Melts. *National Geographic.* April 18, 2019. *www.nationalgeographic.com/environment/2019/04/himalayan-glacial-lakes-threaten-flash-floods-ice-dams-melt-tibetan-plateau*

15. Case A, Deaton A. Mortality and Morbidity in the 21st Century. Brookings Papers on Economic Activity, Spring 2017. *https://scholar.princeton.edu/accase/publications/mortality-and-morbidity-21st-century*

16. World Forum on Natural Capital. *What Is Natural Capital. https://naturalcapitalforum.com/ about.* Accessed November 19, 2019.

17. Krugman P. Despair, American Style. *The New York Times.* November 9, 2015. *www.nytimes. com/2015/11/09/opinion/despair-american-style.html*

18. Raworth K. How Can We Create a Thriving Economy for Ourselves and the Planet? Interview with Guy Raz, National Public Radio, December 7, 2018. *www.npr.org/templates/ transcript/transcript.php?storyId=674117856*

19. Raworth K. *Doughnut Economics: Seven Ways to Think Like a 21st-Century Economist,* 2017, Chelsea Green Publishing; 2017. Cited in *What I Learned This Week,* April 13, 2017, 13D Research, *https://latest.13d.com/instead-of-economies-that-make-us-grow-we-need-economies-that-make-us-thrive-ceec2760bb6a*

Chapter 7

(**References Provided by Author.**)

1. Brand FS, Jax K. Focusing the Meaning(s) of Resilience: Resilience as a Descriptive Concept and a Boundary Object. *Ecology and Society*. 2007;12(1):23. *www.ecologyandsociety.org/vol12/iss1/art23/*. Accessed October 12, 2019.

2. Bond C, Strong A, Burger N, Weilant S, Saya U, Chandra A. (2017). Resilience Dividend Valuation Model: Framework Development and Initial Case Studies. Santa Monica, CA: RAND Corporation. *www.rand.org/pubs/research_reports/RR2129.html*. Accessed October 12, 2019.

3. City of Pittsburgh. OnePGH website. *www.pittsburghpa.gov/onepgh/*. Accessed October 12, 2019.

4. Abramson DM, Grattan LM, Mayer B, et al. The Resilience Activation Framework: A Conceptual Model of How Access to Social Resources Promotes Adaptation and Rapid Recovery in Post-Disaster Settings. *Journal of Behavioral Health Services & Research*. 2015;42(1):42–57.

5. Masten AS, Best KM, Garmezy N. Resilience and Development: Contributions from the Study of Children Who Overcome Adversity. *Development and Psychopathology*. 1990;2(04):425–444.

6. Chandra A, Acosta JD, Howard S, et al. Building Community Resilience to Disasters: A Way Forward to Enhance National Health Security. Santa Monica, CA: RAND Corporation, 2011. www.rand.org/pubs/technical_reports/TR915.html.

7. Cutter SL, Barnes L, Berry M, et al. A Place-Based Model for Understanding Community Resilience to Natural Disasters. *Global Environmental Change*. 2008;18:598–606.

8. Cutter SL, Boruff BJ, Shirley WL. Social Vulnerability to Environmental Hazards. *Social Science Quarterly*. 2003;84(2):242–261.

9. Bruneau M, Chang SE, Eguchi RT, et al. A Framework to Quantitatively Assess and Enhance the Seismic Resilience of Communities. *Earthquake Spectra*. 2003;19(4):733–752.

10. Brodie M, Weltzien E, Altman D, Blendon RJ, Benson JM. Experiences of Hurricane Katrina Evacuees in Houston Shelters: Implications for Future Planning. *American Journal of Public Health*. 2006;96(8):1402–1408.

11. Carpenter SR, Folke C, Norstrom A, et al. Program on Ecosystem Change and Society: An International Research Strategy for Integrated Social-Ecological Systems. *Current Opinion in Environmental Sustainability*. 2012;4:134–138.

12. Calhoun LG, Tedeschi RG. Posttraumatic Growth: Future Directions. In: Tedeschi RG, Calhoun LG, eds. *Posttraumatic Growth: Positive Changes in the Aftermath of Crisis*. Mahwah, NJ: Lawrence Erlbaum Associates; 1998;215–238.

13. Zatura A, Hall J, Murray K. Community Development and Community Resilience: An Integrative Approach. *Community Development*. 2009;39(3):130–147.

14. City of Santa Monica. Office of Civic Wellbeing website. *wellbeing.smgov.net*. Accessed October 12, 2019.

15. Shelton T, Zook M, Wiig A. The "Actually Existing Smart City." *Cambridge Journal of Regions, Economy and Society*. 2015;8(1):13–25.

16. Chun SA, Shulman S, Sandoval Almazan R, Hovy E. Government 2.0: Making Connections Between Citizens, Data and Government. *Information Polity*. 2010;15(1,2):1–9.

17. Acosta J, Chandra A, Madrigano J. (2017). An Agenda to Advance Integrative Resilience Research and Practice. RAND Corporation. Santa Monica, CA. *www.rand.org/pubs/research_reports/RR1683.html*

18. O'Brien K, Hayward B, Berkes F. Rethinking social contracts: building resilience in a changing climate. *Ecology and Society*. 2009;14(2):12. *www.ecologyandsociety.org/vol14/iss2/art12/*. Accessed October 12, 2019.

19. FEMA. (2018). Disaster Declarations. *www.fema.gov/disasters*

20. Calderón-Contreras R, White CS. Access as the Means for Understanding Social-Ecological Resilience: Bridging Analytical Frameworks. *Society & Natural Resources.* 2019:1–19. *DOI: 10.1080/08941920.2019.1597233.*

21. National Academy of Sciences. (2015). Measures of Community Resilience for Local Decision Makers. Proceedings of a Workshop. Washington, D.C.: National Academies Press.

22. Asadzadeh A, Kötter T, Salehi P, Birkmann J. Operationalizing a Concept: The Systematic Review of Composite Indicator Building for Measuring Community Disaster Resilience. *International Journal of Disaster Risk Reduction.* 2017;25:147–162.

23. Fiskel J. Sustainability and Resilience: Towards a Systems Approach. *Sustainability: Science, Practice & Policy.* 2006;2:14–21.

24. Archer D, Dodman D. Making Capacity Building Critical: Power and Justice in Building Urban Climate Resilience in Indonesia and Thailand. *Urban Climate.* 2015;14(Part 1):68–78.

25. Fois F, Forino G. The Self-Built Ecovillage in L'Aquila, Italy: Community Resilience as a Grassroots Response to Environmental Shock. *Disasters.* 2014;38(4):719–739.

26. Colding J, Barthel S. The Potential of "Urban Green Commons" in the Resilience Building of Cities. *Ecological Economics.* 2013;86:156–166.

27. North P, Longhurst N. Grassroots localisation? The Scalar Potential of and Limits of the "Transition" Approach to Climate Change and Resource Constraint. *Urban Studies.* 2013;50(7):1423–1438.

28. Norris FH, Stevens SP, Pfefferbaum B, Wyche KF, Pfefferbaum RL. Community Resilience as a Metaphor, Theory, Set of Capacities, and Strategy for Disaster Readiness. *American Journal of Community Psychology.* 2008;41(1–2);127–150.

29. Walker J, Cooper M. Genealogies of Resilience: From Systems Ecology to the Political Economy of Crisis Adaptation. *Security Dialogue.* 2011;42(2):143–160. *doi.org/10.1177/0967010611399616.* Accessed October 12, 2019.

30. Wendell J. Complex Adaptive Systems. 2003. Beyond Intractability, Conflict Research Consortium Website. *www.beyondintractability.org/essay/complex_adaptive_systems.* Accessed October 12, 2019.

31. Ungar M, Ghazinour M, Richter J. Annual Research Review: What is Resilience Within the Social Ecology of Human Development? *Journal of Child Psychology and Psychiatry.* 2013;54(4):348–366.

32. Zolkoski SM, Bullock LM. Resilience in Children and Youth: A Review. *Children and Youth Services Review.* 2012;34(12):2295–2303.

33. Aldrich DP. *Building resilience: Social Capital in Post-Disaster Recovery.* Chicago: University of Chicago Press; 2012.

34. Aldrich DP, Meyer MA. Social Capital and Community Resilience. *American Behavioral Scientist.* 2015;59(2):254–269.

35. Matin N, Forrester J, Ensor J. What Is Equitable Resilience? *World Development.* 2018;109:197–205.

36. Davoudi S, Shaw K, Haider JL, et al. Resilience: A Bridging Concept or a Dead End? "Reframing" Resilience: Challenges for Planning Theory and Practice. *Planning Theory & Practice.* 2012;13(2):299–333.

37. Tzoulas K, Korpela K, Venn S, et al. Promoting Ecosystem and Human Health in Urban areas using Green Infrastructure: A Literature Review. *Landscape and Urban Planning.* 2007;81(3):167–178.

38. Colvin HM, Taylor RM. Five Resilience Programs and Interventions. Building a Resilient Workforce: Opportunities for the Department of Homeland Security: Workshop Summary. Washington, D.C.: National Academies Press; 2012.

39. Brown TM, Fee E. Social Movements in Health. *Annual Review of Public Health.* 2014;35:385–398.

40. Shankardass K, Muntaner C, Kokkinen L, et al. The Implementation of Health in All Policies Initiatives: A Systems Framework for Government Action. *Health Research Policy and Systems.* 2018;16(1):26.

41. Hoffman B. Health Care Reform and Social Movements in the United States. *American Journal of Public Health.* 2003;93(1):75–85.

42. Kapilashrami A, Smith KE, Fustukian S, et al. Social Movements and Public Health Advocacy in Action: The UK People's Health Movement. *Journal of Public Health.* 2016;38(3):413–416.

43. de Camargo KR, Jr. Democratic Policy, Social Movements, and Public Health: A New Theme for AJPH Public Health Forum. *American Journal of Public Health.* 2017;107(12):1855–1856.

44. Barr S. Helping People Make Better Choices: Exploring the Behaviour Change Agenda for Environmental Sustainability. *Applied Geography (Sevenoaks).* 2011;31(2):712–720.

45. McKenzie S. Social Sustainability: Towards Some Definitions. Working Paper Series No. 27. Magill, Australia: University of South Australia, Hawke Research Institute; 2004.

46. Hawkins CA. Building Bridges and Crossing Boundaries: Critical Connections for Contemporary Social Work. *Critical Social Work.* 2010;11(3).

47. Epstein MJ, Roy M. Making the Business Case for Sustainability: Linking Social and Environmental Actions to Financial Performance. *Journal of Corporate Citizenship.* 2003;Spring:79–95.

48. Atkinson S, Bagnall AM, Corcoran R, et al. (2017). *What is Community Wellbeing? Conceptual Review.* What Works Centre for Wellbeing. *whatworkswellbeing.org/product/ what-is-community-wellbeing-conceptual-review/.* Accessed October 12, 2019.

49. Lemos MC, Agrawal A. Environmental Governance. *Annual Review of Environment and Natural Resources.* 2006;31:297–325.

50. Abdallah S. (2013). Considerations for Well-Being Measurement in Santa Monica.

51. Forgeard MJC, Jayawickreme E, Kern M, Seligman MEP. Doing the Right Thing: Measuring Wellbeing for Public Policy. *International Journal of Wellbeing.* 2011;1(1):79–106.

52. Kahneman D, Kruger D, et al. A Survey Method for Characterizing Daily Life Experience. *Science.* 2004;306:1776–1780.

53. Abdallah S, Thompson S, Michaelson J, Marks N, Steuer N. The (un)Happy Planet Index 2.0: Why Good Lives Don't Have to Cost the Earth. London: New Economics Foundation; 2009.

54. New Zealand Government. The Wellbeing Budget 2019. The Treasury website. *treasury. govt. nz/publications/wellbeing-budget/wellbeing-budget-2019-html.* Accessed October 12, 2019.

55. Baezconde-Garbanati L, Unger J, Portugal C, Delgado JL, Falcon A, Gaitan M. Maximizing Participation of Hispanic Community-Based/Non-Governmental Organizations (NGOs) in Emergency Preparedness. *International Quarterly of Community Health Education.* 2006;24(4):289–317.

56. Pant AT, Kirsch TD, Subbarao IR, Hsieh Y-H, Vu A. Faith-Based Organizations and Sustainable Sheltering Operations in Mississippi after Hurricane Katrina: Implications for Informal Network Utilization. *Prehospital and Disaster Medicine.* 2008;23(1):48–54.

57. Stewart GT, Kolluru R, Smith M. Leveraging Public-Private Partnerships to Improve Community Resilience. *International Journal of Physical Distribution and Logistics Management.* 2009;39(5):343–364.

58. Mechanic D, Tanner J. Vulnerable People, Groups, and Populations: Societal View. *Health Affairs.* 2007;26(5):1220–1230.

59. Morrow BH. Identifying and Mapping Community Vulnerability. *Disasters.* 1999;23(1):1–18.

60. Pfefferbaum BJ, Pfefferbaum RL, Norris FH. Community Resilience and Wellness for Children Exposed to Hurricane Katrina. In: Kilmer RP, Gil-Rivas V, Tedeschi RG, Calhoun LG, eds. *Helping Families and Communities Recover from Disaster: Lessons Learned from Hurricane Katrina and Its Aftermath.* Washington, D.C.: American Psychological Association; 2009:265–288.

61. Holt-Lunstad J, Smith TB, Baker M, Harris T, Stephenson D. Loneliness and Social Isolation as Risk Factors for Mortality: A Meta-Analytic Review. *Perspectives on Psychological Science.* 2015;10(2):227–237.

62. Cigna. U.S. Loneliness Index. 2018. *www.cigna.com/assets/docs/newsroom/loneliness-survey-2018-full-report.pdf.* Accessed October 12, 2019.

63. Varda DM, Chandra A, Stern SA, Lurie N. Core Dimensions of Connectivity in Public Health Collaboratives. *Journal of Public Health Management and Practice.* 2008;14(5):E1–E7.

64. Kim YC, Kang J. Communication, Neighbourhood Belonging and Household Hurricane Preparedness. *Disasters.* 2010;34(2):470–488.

65. McMillan DW, Chavis DM. Sense of Community: A Definition and Theory. *Journal of Community Psychology.* 1986;14(1):6–23.

66. Kailes JI, Enders A. Moving Beyond "Special Needs": A Function-Based Framework for Emergency Management and Planning. *Journal of Disability Policy Studies.* 2007;17(4):230–237.

67. Chandra A, Cahill M, Yeung D, Ross R. *Toward an Initial Conceptual Framework to Assess Community Allostatic Load: Early Themes from Literature Review and Community Analyses on the Role of Cumulative Community Stress.* Santa Monica, CA: RAND Corporation; 2018. *https://www.rand.org/pubs/research_reports/RR2559.html*

68. Hess P, Moudon A, Snyder M, et al. Site Design and Pedestrian Travel. *Transportation Research Record: Journal of the Transportation Research Board.* 1999;1674:9–19.

69. Moudon A, Hess P, Snyder M, et al. Effects of Site Design on Pedestrian Travel in Mixed-Use, Medium Density Environments. *Transportation Research Record: Journal of the Transportation Research Board.* 1997;1578:48–55.

70. Bellanca JA, Brandt R, eds. *21st Century Skills: Rethinking How Students Learn.* Bloomington, IN: Solution Tree Press; 2010.

Chapter 9

(**References Provided by Author.**)

1. Ardern J. *Prime Minister Jacinda Ardern's Wellbeing Budget Speech.* May 30, 2019.

2. The Treasury. *Our People, Our Country, Our Future: Living Standards Framework: Background and Future Work.* December 4, 2018.

3. Gleisner B, McAlister F, Galt M, Beaglehole J. A Living Standards Approach to Public Policy Making. *New Zealand Economic Papers.* 2012;46(3):211.

4. Robeyns I. The Capability Approach. In: *The Stanford Encyclopedia of Philosophy (Winter 2016 Edition),* Edward N. Zalta, ed. *https:// plato.stanford.edu/ archives/ win2016/ entries/ capability- approach/*

5. Fleurbaey M. Beyond GDP: The Quest for a Measure of Social Welfare. *Journal of Economic Literature.* 2009;47(4):1029–1075.

6. Stiglitz J, Sen A, Fitoussi J-P. (2009, September). *Report by the Commission on the Measurement of Economic Performance and Social Progress.*

7. Briassoulis H. *Policy Integration for Complex Policy Problems: What, Why and How.* Paper presented for the conference "Greening of Policies: Interlinkages and Policy Integration," Berlin, 2004.

8. Candel J, Biesbroek R. Toward a Processual Understanding of Policy Integration. *Policy Science.* 2016;49:211–231.

9. Senik C. Wealth and Happiness. *Oxford Review of Economic Policy.* 2014;30(1): 92–108.

10. Durand M, Exton C. (2019). Adopting a Wellbeing Approach in Central Government: Policy Mechanisms and Practical Tools. In: Global Happiness Council, *Global Happiness and Wellbeing Policy Report,* Ch. 8.

11. Lange G, Wodon Q, Carey K. *The Changing Wealth of Nations 2018: Building a Sustainable Future.* World Bank Group; 2018.

12. Exton C, Shinwell M. (2018). Policy Use of Well-Being Metrics: Describing Countries' Experiences. OECD: SDD Working Paper No. 94.

13. Durand M. (2018). Countries' Experiences with Wellbeing and Happiness Metrics. In Global Happiness Council, *Global Happiness Report,* Ch. 8.

14. Robertson G. *Minister of Finance Wellbeing Budget Speech.* May 30, 2019.

15. Shrikanth S. NZ Unveils "Wellbeing" Budget as Economy Slows. *Financial Times,* May 29, 2019.

16. Ainge Roy E. New Zealand "Wellbeing" Budget Promises Billions to Care for Most Vulnerable. *The Guardian*, May 30, 2019.

17. Rondinella T. Policy Use of ProgressI. In: Rondinella T, Signore M, Fazio D, Grazia Calza M, Righi A, eds. *Map on Policy Use of Progress Indicators*. Istat; June 2014.

18. Scarre G. *Utilitarianism*. Routledge; 2002.

19. O'Connell E, Greenaway T, Moeke T, McMeeking S. (2018). He Ara Waiora: A Pathway towards Wellbeing. *New Zealand Treasury Discussion Paper*, 18/11.

20. Te Puni Kōkiri and The Treasury. (2019, January). An Indigenous Approach to the Living Standards Framework. *Treasury Discussion Paper*, 19/01.

21. Thomsen S, Tavita J, Levi-Teu Z. (2018, August). A Pacific Perspective on the Living Standards Framework and Wellbeing. *Treasury Discussion Paper*, 18/09.

22. Yong S. (2018, September). An Asian Perspective and the New Zealand Treasury Living Standards Framework. *Treasury Discussion Paper*, 18/10.

23. Dalziel P, Saunders C, Savage C. (2019, June). Culture, Wellbeing, and the Living Standards Framework: A Perspective. *Treasury Discussion Paper*, 19/02.

24. Smith C. *Treasury Living Standards Dashboard: Monitoring Intergenerational Wellbeing*. Kōtātā Insight; 2018.

25. King A, Huseynli G, MacGibbon N. (2018, February). Wellbeing Frameworks for the Treasury. *Treasury Living Standards Series: Discussion Paper*, 18/01.

26. The Treasury. (2016, November). Conversations about Things That Matter: Reflections from the Treasury's Long-Term Fiscal Statement External Engagement Process.

27. Te Rito J, ed. Mātauranga Taketake: Traditional Knowledge: Indigenous Indicators of Well-Being: Perspectives, Practices, Solutions. Conference Proceedings. Ngā Pae o te Māramatanga: The National Institute of Research Excellence for Māori Development and Advancement, Wellington, June 14–17, 2006.

28. OECD. (2019, June 25). *OECD Economic Surveys: New Zealand 2019*.

29. The Treasury. CBAx Tool User Guidance: Guide for Departments and Agencies Using Treasury's CBAx Tool for Cost Benefit Analysis. September 2018.

30. English W. Speech to the Treasury Guest Lecture Series on Social Investment. September 18, 2015.

31. Robertson G. (2017, December 14). Budget Policy Statement 2018. New Zealand Government.

32. Labour Party. (2017). *Labour's Fiscal Plan: Post PREFU Revision*.

33. Robertson G. Speech to the Institute of Public Administration New Zealand (IPANZ). February 15, 2018.

34. OECD. (2019). Policy Coherence for Sustainable Development 2019: Empowering People and Ensuring Inclusiveness and Equality, 14.

35. The Treasury. (2014). Holding On and Letting Go: Opportunities and Challenges for New Zealand's Economic Performance.

36. The Treasury. (2016). *He Tirohanga Mokopuna*: 2016 Statement on the Long-Term Fiscal Position.

37. The Treasury. (2018). *He Puna Hao Pātiki*: 2018 Investment Statement: Investing for Wellbeing.

38. Te Puni Kōkiri. (2016). The Whānau Ora Outcomes Framework: Empowering Whānau into the Future.

39. New Zealand Government. (2018). *Government Policy Statement on Land Transport, 2018/19-2027/28*.

40. Ardern J. *Speech from the Throne*. November 8, 2017.

41. The Treasury. (2018, September 19). *Budget 2019: Guidance for Agencies*.

42. New Zealand Government. (2019, May 30). *Budget 2019: The Wellbeing Budget*.

43. The Treasury. (2019, August). *Better Business Cases*.

44. The Treasury. (2015, July). *Guide to Social Cost Benefit Analysis*.

45. Räsänen P, Roine E, Sintonen H, Semberg-Konttinen V, Ryynänen O, Roine, R. Use of Quality-Adjusted Life Years for the Estimation of Effectiveness of Health Care: A Systematic Literature Review. *International Journal of Technology Assessment in Health Care.* 2006;22(2):235.

46. Ministry of Education. (2017, April). Track 1 Initiative Template: Vote Education—Early Identification and Removal of Communication Barriers to the Curriculum. *https://treasury.govt. nz/publications/information-release/applied-examples-cbax-budget-2017-information-release*

47. Ministry of Justice. (2017, July). Track 1 Initiative Template: Track 1 Investment Approach to Justice: Reducing Youth Offending. *https:// treasury.govt.nz/publications/information-release/applied-examples-cbax-budget-2017-information-release*

48. Scott R, Boyd R. (2017). Interagency Performance Targets: A Case Study of New Zealand's Results Programme. IBM Center for the Business of Government.

49. Arnaboldi M, Lapsley I, Steccolini I. Performance Management in the Public Sector: The Ultimate Challenge. *Financial Accountability & Management.* 2015;31(1):1–22.

50. Diefenbach T. New Public Management in Public Sector Organisations: The Dark Sides of Managerialistic "Enlightenment." *Public Administration.* 2009;87(4):892–909.

51. Kurtz C, Snowden D. The New Dynamics of Strategy: Sense-Making in a Complex and Complicated World. *IBM Systems Journal.* 2003;42(3):462.

52. Westley F, Antadze N. Making a Difference: Strategies for Scaling Social Innovation for Greater Impact. *Innovation Journal.* 2010;15(2):article 2.

53. Howlett M, Rayner J. Design Principles for Policy Mixes: Cohesion and Coherence in "New Governance Arrangements." *Policy and Society.* 2007;26(4):1.

54. New Zealand Productivity Commission. (2015, August). More Effective Social Services.

55. Waikato Regional Council. (2017, May). Waikato Progress Indicators—Tupuranga Waikato: Summary Update. *Waikato Regional Council Technical Report.* 2017/16.

56. Johnson A. (2018, February). Kei a Tātou: It Is Us: State of the Nation Report. The Salvation Army Social Policy & Parliamentary Unit.

57. Lucas D, Kelly J. (2018). Inclusive and Resilient Communities: Co-Creating Our Human and Social Capital. *State of the State,* Article 5, Deloitte.

58. Social Investment Agency. *Social Investment Agency's Beginners' Guide to the Integrated Data Infrastructure.* Wellington, N.Z.; 2017.

59. Gruen N. Nicholas Gruen: What Have Wellbeing Frameworks Ever Done for Us? *The Mandarin,* October 18, 2017.

60. Gruen N. Nicholas Gruen: Hacking Wellbeing for the Biggest Returns. *The Mandarin,* October 19, 2017.

61. Dann L. Big Read: Treasury's Bold New Plan to Measure Your Well-Being. *New Zealand Herald,* April 5, 2018.

62. Grimes A. NZ Policy from a Wellbeing Perspective. *Newsroom,* July 3, 2017.

63. Wilkinson B. (2016). Treasury's Living Standards Framework. *Asymmetric Information 55.* New Zealand Association of Economists, 7.

64. Reddell M. The Treasury Reminds Us That GDP—and Productivity—Really Is Almost Everything. *Croaking Cassandra,* March 10, 2018.

Chapter 10

1. Schaffer J. UN's Sustainable Development Goals Positively Influence Impact Investing. June 7, 2017. *https://nonprofitquarterly.org/uns-sustainable-development-goals-positively-influence-impact-investing/.* Accessed October 18, 2019.

2. Sustainable Development Goal 3. United Nations website. *https://sustainabledevelopment.un.org/sdg3*. Accessed October 18, 2019.

3. Feloni R. BlackRock CEO Larry Fink Says within the Next 5 Years All Investors Will Measure a Company's Impact on Society, Government, and the Environment to Determine Its Worth. Business Insider. November 1, 2018. *businessinsider.com/blackrock-larry-fink-investors-esg-metrics-2018-11*. Accessed October 18, 2019.

4. Durand M, Exton C. (2019). Adopting a Well-Being Approach in Central Government: Policy Mechanisms and Practical Tools. In: Global Happiness Council, *Global Happiness and Well-Being Policy Report*. Chapter 8.

5. Wallace J. *Wellbeing and Devolution: Reframing the Role of Government in Scotland, Wales and Northern Ireland*. London: Palgrave Pivot; 2019.

Afterword: The Future of Well-Being

1. Sartorius N. The Meanings of Health and Its Promotion. *Croatian Medical Journal*. 2006;47(4):662–664.

2. Lloyd-Jones DM, Hong Y, Labarthe D, et al. Defining and Setting National Goals for Cardiovascular Health Promotion and Disease Reduction: The American Heart Association's Strategic Impact Goal through 2020 and Beyond. *Circulation*. 2010;121(4):586–613.

3. Labarthe DR, Kubzansky LD, Boehm JK, Lloyd-Jones DM, Berry JD, Seligman ME. Positive Cardiovascular Health: A Timely Convergence. *Journal of the American College of Cardiology*. 2016;68(8):860–867.

4. Kubzansky LD, Segerstrom SC, Boehm JK. Positive Psychological Functioning and the Biology of Health. *Social and Personality Psychology Compass*. 2015;9(12):645–660.

5. Farrelly C. "Positive biology" as a New Paradigm for the Medical Sciences. Focusing on People Who Live Long, Happy, Healthy Lives Might Hold the Key to Improving Human Well-Being. *EMBO Reports*. 2012;13(3):186–188.

6. VanderWeele TJ, Chen Y, Long KN, Kim ES, Trudel-Fitzgerald C, Kubzansky LD. Positive Epidemiology? *Epidemiology*. 2020;31(2):189–193.

7. Pressman SD, Jenkins BN, Moskowitz JT. Positive Affect and Health: What Do We Know and Where Next Should We Go? *Annual Review of Psychology*. 2019;70:627–650.

8. Steptoe A. Happiness and Health. *Annual Review of Public Health*. 2019;40:339–359.

9. Boehm JK, Chen Y, Koga H, Mathur MB, Vie LL, Kubzansky LD. Is Optimism Associated with Healthier Cardiovascular-Related Behavior? Meta-Analyses of 3 Health Behaviors. *Circulation Research*. 2018;122(8):1119–1134.

10. Boehm JK, Soo J, Zevon ES, Chen Y, Kim ES, Kubzansky LD. Longitudinal Associations between Psychological Well-Being and the Consumption of Fruits and Vegetables. *Health Psychology*. 2018;37(10):959–967.

11. Kim ES, Kubzansky LD, Soo J, Boehm JK. Maintaining Healthy Behavior: A Prospective Study of Psychological Well-Being and Physical Activity. *Annals of Behavioral Medicine*. 2017;51(3):337–347.

12. Cameron DS, Bertenshaw EJ, Sheeran P. Positive Affect and Physical Activity: Testing Effects on Goal Setting, Activation, Prioritisation, and Attainment. *Psychology and Health*. 2018;33(2):258–274.

13. Steptoe A, Wardle J. Positive Affect and Biological Function in Everyday Life. *Neurobiology of Aging*. 2005;26 Suppl 1:108–112.

14. Steptoe A, Wardle J. Life Skills, Wealth, Health, and Wellbeing in Later Life. *Proceedings of the National Academy of Science of the United States of America*. 2017;114(17):4354–4359.

15. Huffman JC, Millstein RA, Mastromauro CA, et al. A Positive Psychology Intervention for Patients with an Acute Coronary Syndrome: Treatment Development and Proof-of-Concept Trial. *Journal of Happiness Studies*. 2016;17(5):1985–2006.

16. Peterson JC, Charlson ME, Hoffman Z, et al. A Randomized Controlled Trial of Positive-Affect Induction to Promote Physical Activity after Percutaneous Coronary Intervention. *Archives of Internal Medicine*. 2012;172(4):329–336.

17. Kossek EE, Thompson RJ, Lawson KM, et al. Caring for the Elderly at Work and Home: Can a Randomized Organizational Intervention Improve Psychological Health? *Journal of Occupational Health Psychology*. 2019;24(1):36–54.

18. Thornton RLJ, Glover CM, Cené CW, Glik DC, Henderson JA, Williams DR. Evaluating Strategies for Reducing Health Disparities by Addressing the Social Determinants of Health. *Health Affairs*. 2016;35(8):1416–1423.

19. Berkman LF. Social Epidemiology: Social Determinants of Health in the United States: Are We Losing Ground? *Annual Review of Public Health*. 2009;30:27–41.

20. Plough AL. Building a Culture of Health: A Critical Role for Public Health Services and Systems Research. *American Journal of Public Health*. 2015;105(Suppl 2):S150–S152.

21. United Nations Development Programme. Human Development Index (HDI). United Nations Development Programme, Human Development Reports, 2018. *http://hdr.undp. org/en/content/human-development-index-hdi*. Accessed January 20, 2019.

22. Stiglitz JE, Sen AK, Fitoussi JP. (2009). *Report by the Commission on the Measurement of Economic Performance and Social Progress*. Paris. *https://ec.europa.eu/eurostat/documents/ 118025/118123/Fitoussi+Commission+report*

23. Syme SL. Foreword to the second edition of *Social Epidemiology*. In: Berkman LF, Kawachi I, Glymour MM, eds. *Social Epidemiology*. Oxford: Oxford University Press; 2014, vii–x.

24. Bradshaw J, Martorano B, Natali L, De Neubourg C. Children's Subjective Well-Being in Rich Countries. *Child Indicators Research*. 2013;6:619–635.

25. Su R, Tay L, Diener E. The Development and Validation of the Comprehensive Inventory of Thriving (CIT) and the Brief Inventory of Thriving (BIT). *Applied Psychology Health and Well-Being*. 2014;6(3):251–279.

26. National Research Council. *Subjective Well-Being: Measuring Happiness, Suffering, and Other Dimensions of Experience*. Washington, DC: The National Academies Press; 2013.

27. Organisation for Economic Cooperation and Development. (2013). OECD Guidelines on Measuring Subjective Well-Being.

28. VanderWeele TJ, Trudel-Fitzgerald C, Allin P, et al. Current Recommendations on the Selection of Measures for Well-Being. In: Lee M, Kubzansky LD, VanderWeele TJ, eds. *Measuring Well-Being: Interdisciplinary Perspectives from the Social Sciences and the Humanities*. New York: Oxford University Press; forthcoming.

29. Ravens-Sieberer U, Devine J, Bevans K, et al. Subjective Well-Being Measures for Children Were Developed within the PROMIS Project: Presentation of First Results. *Journal of Clinical Epidemiology*. 2014;67(2):207–218.

30. Boehm JK, Kim ES, Kubzansky LD. Positive Psychological Well-Being. In: Kivimaki M, Batty D, Steptoe A, Kawachi I, eds. *The Routledge International Handbook of Psychosocial Epidemiology*. New York: Routledge; 2018:156–169.

31. Helliwell J, Layard R, Sachs J. *World Happiness Report*. New York; 2017.

32. Cohen S. Social Relationships and Health. *American Psychologist*. 2004;59(8):676–684.

33. Helgeson VS, Cohen S, Schulz R, Yasko J. Group Support Interventions for Women with Breast Cancer: Who Benefits from What? *Health Psychology*. 2000;19(2):107–114.

34. Weinstein N, Ryan RM. When Helping Helps: Autonomous Motivation for Prosocial Behavior and Its Influence on Well-Being for the Helper and Recipient. *Journal of Personality and Social Psychology*. 2010;98(2):222–244.

35. Robert Wood Johnson Foundation. (2019). *Building a Culture of Health: Why We Need a Culture of Health*. *www.rwjf.org/en/cultureofhealth/about/why-we-need-a-culture-of-health. html*. Accessed December 9, 2019.

Afterword: A Vision for Well-Being Policies and Action in the United States, Based on Santa Monica's Experience

1. Raposa EB, Rhodes J, Stams GJJM, et al. The Effects of Youth Mentoring Programs: A Meta-Analysis of Outcome Studies. *Journal of Youth and Adolescence.* 2019;48(3):4230443.
2. Spencer R, Gowdy G, Drew AL, Rhodes JE. Who Knows Me the Best and Can Encourage Me the Most?: Matching and Early Relationships Development in Youth-Initiated Mentoring Relationships with System-Involved Youth. *Journal of Adolescent Research.* 2019;34(1):3–29.

Conclusion

1. Iceland Puts Well-Being Ahead of GDP in Budget. *BBC News.* December 3, 2019. *www.bbc com/news/world-europe-50650155*
2. Charlton E. New Zealand Has Unveiled Its First "Well-Being" Budget. World Economic Forum. *www.weforum.org/agenda/2019/05/new-zealand-is-publishing-its-first-well-being-budget.* Accessed January 15, 2020.
3. Sturgeon N. *Why governments should prioritize well-being.* TED Summit, July 2019. *www.ted. com/talks/nicola_sturgeon_why_governments_should_prioritize_   well_being?language=en.* Accessed January 15, 2020.
4. Partington, R. Wellbeing Should Replace Growth as "Main Aim of UK Spending." *The Guardian.* May 23, 2019. *www.theguardian.com/politics/2019/may/24/ wellbeing-should-replace-growth-as-main-aim-of-uk-spending*
5. Woolf SH, Schoomaker H. Life Expectancy and Mortality Rates in the United States, 1959–2017. *JAMA.* 2019;322(20):1996–2016.

INDEX